Yoga
for Osteoporosis

Yoga
for Osteoporosis

The Complete Guide

Loren Fishman, MD
Ellen Saltonstall

W. W. Norton & Company
New York • London

For information about permission to reproduce selections from this book,
write to Permissions, W. W. Norton & Company, Inc.,
500 Fifth Avenue, New York, NY 10110

For information about special discounts for bulk purchases, please contact
W. W. Norton Special Sales at specialsales@wwnorton.com or 800-233-4830

Manufacturing by Courier Westford
Book design by Molly Heron
Production manager: Devon Zahn

Library of Congress Cataloging-in-Publication Data

Fishman, Loren.
Yoga for osteoporosis : the complete guide / Loren Fishman, Ellen Saltonstall.
p. cm.
Includes bibliographical references and index.
ISBN 978-0-393-33485-2 (pbk.)
1. Osteoporosis—Exercise therapy. 2. Yoga—Therapeutic use. I. Saltonstall, Ellen. II. Title.
RC931.O73F57 2010
616.7'160642—dc22
2009025384

W. W. Norton & Company, Inc.
500 Fifth Avenue, New York, N.Y. 10110
www.wwnorton.com

W. W. Norton & Company Ltd.
Castle House, 75 / 76 Wells Street, London W1T 3QT

2 3 4 5 6 7 8 9 0

To our teachers,
and all teachers and therapists using
HEALTHFUL *means to improve health.*

Contents

List of Illustrations

Acknowledgments

The authors would like to thank B. K. S. Iyengar and John Friend for their wisdom, astute precepts, and examples, and Krishnamacharya for the tradition in which so many of our teachers stand. We are extremely grateful to Tommy Moorman for his fine hand and patience in creating numerous illustrations and their numberless reincarnations in this book and in *Yoga for Arthritis*. We also thank Donal Holway and Julio Torres for excellent photography, Susan Genis and David Fink for remarkable guidance during the photo shoots, and Sally Hess and Rachel Fishman for their expert modeling and support. We thank our editors at W. W. Norton—Jill Bialosky, Evan Carver, Paul Whitlatch, Adrienne Davich, Alison Liss, and Kristin Sperber—both for making the manuscript more intelligible and for understanding us. Once again we thank Carol Stratten, Dr. David Palmieri, and Norman Brettler of Dynamic Imaging in Tilton, New Jersey, for their generous donation of time and facilities that made dynamic MRI studies of yoga possible.

Thanks to our students and patients for the many elucidating exchanges that have occurred in the process of yoga therapy; for their personal improvement they must thank themselves. Last and most overdue, we acknowledge a debt to our families for their willing sacrifices during the periods of writing and revision.

Authors' Note

Scientists and healers enjoy certain "rights of access": We can enter our patients' personal space, ask intimate questions, and give advice that, subject to the sacred sieve of scientific skepticism, is generally taken seriously. Our rights are earned through a combination of aptitude, study, and personal trust.

But scientists and healers only exist within the complex matrix of their society, and along with their rights come certain responsibilities. Among those responsibilities are impartial seeking and sharing of the truth, articulately and intelligibly responding to problems, questioning what is seen as unwise practice or false belief, and selfless giving of help when and where it is needed. Yet national security and commercial confidentiality often require that scientists *not* share all information. Healers also have legally delimited confidentiality and may choose not to vitiate their gift by disseminating what is, by necessity, only part of the story. This censorship, self-imposed or otherwise, is consistent with the society-wide duty to share what one knows only if the sharing and use of the knowledge are equally discreet. Please use the information herein with humble awareness of the vast present and future human experience of which it forms a very small part.

In the healing arts a commitment to open communication must be tempered by caution. On the societal level, just as with individuals, scientists and healers have a responsibility to "do no harm." Here yoga therapy leads the way. The flow and structure of what is known about yoga survives only through mutual trust, as much among those who want to know as those who know already. Being passed on from individual to individual, it nevertheless has societal aims: peace and thoughtfulness. The morality is part of the message.

There is another general problem that yoga therapy resolves rather gracefully: All the healing arts must synthesize abstract and anonymous laws of biology to accommodate individuals' needs and vulnerabilities. If we just adhere to the general laws of science, individual uniqueness falls out of the equation. But if we only attend to an individual's circumstances, treatment is merely anecdotal, and the vast legacy of scientific fact is ignored. Healers are able to heal when patients trust them to adjust and apply objective laws to the advantage of the individual's particular case. This trust is what makes medical science practical and most healing possible. Yogis have been earning this trust for thousands of years.

We hope that yoga will appeal to people of all ages; we know that osteoporosis is most effectively countered in the teens and early twenties! But we expect that many people reading these words will be older, and then another consideration is relevant: the fragility of the bones, joints, and sinews. As you get beyond age 50, some experts look at the facts about mechanoreception and urge "impact" exercise to "stave off bone loss." Unfortunately, another group of experts, with just as much empirical support, caution that impact exercise, such as jogging, can lead rather directly to osteoarthritis.

This puts older people in an impossible position: If they exercise with impact, the bones may stay strong, but the joints at either end will become painful and difficult to move. On the other hand, if they stay away from impact, they will save their joints, but the bones themselves may deteriorate. It's both ends against the middle.

We believe yoga is the answer for older people who want to stay strong, flexible, and pain-free: In yoga the joints are moved to an ever-expanding range, circulating their fluid and stimulating renewal of cartilage, tendons, and ligaments.[1] Simultaneously, the bones are isometrically subjected to forces many times those of gravity, exactly the same forces involved in impact exercise. But in yoga, the forces are applied without any impact—yoga provides an excellent solution to the twin perils of osteoarthritis and osteoporosis.

Yoga

for Osteoporosis

Introduction

D on't want to end your days in a nursing home's wheelchair? Averse to pain? Have little relish for osteonecrosis of the jaw brought on by years of ingesting stomach-upsetting medicines? May we suggest another way? Yoga. Paradoxical as it may seem, yoga—which appears to the uninitiated to be the cessation of outward movement, with its ultimately introspective focus—has in its repertoire the remedy for osteoporosis. We are about to prove this in fine detail.

It would be hard to find a more direct medical application of yoga than to osteoporosis. Bones are strengthened by good diet and sunlight, of course, but that is true of tree trunks too. Force applied to bones stimulates them to grow stronger. The greater the forces applied to a bone, the greater the boney build-up at the point of stress. Wolff's law, which we will come to again in chapters 5 and 6, states that the *architectonic* of bone, its structure, follows the lines of force to which that bone is exposed. Since Wolff's time a persuasive number of studies have shown that, within a bone, levels of different enzymes and biochemical markers of bone synthesis increase abruptly within 10 seconds of adding stress to it. Yoga is a simple, silent, inexpensive, and impact-free way of applying that force exactly as one intends.

Although much research during the past 100 years supports the application of Wolff's law in yoga, this book contains a summary of the first pilot study that actually demonstrates yoga's bone-strengthening benefits. The study also describes an additional advantage for the older person with osteoporosis (as well as osteopenia, the precursor to osteoporosis). The usual prescription for osteoporosis is "weight-bearing and impact exercises." However, most people over 55 have osteoarthritis, and impact exercise is exactly what the rheumatologist did *not* order.

Yoga safely stresses bones without impact, a solution to this dilemma. With many poses that avoid moving joints altogether, yoga has been shown to strengthen bones without any evidence that it weakens joints. On the contrary, several studies find that yoga ameliorates osteoarthritis. Many poses do stretch joint capsules, ligaments, and sinews, moving selected joints through wider ranges of motion. Yoga actually exerts a positive influence on arthritic joints, internally irrigating and moving cartilage-making tissue both within the fluids of the joint and inside the cartilage itself. (For more detail, please see *Yoga for Arthritis*.)

But yoga's advantages do not end there. Almost everyone who practices yoga—including the thousands we have encountered, taught, and treated—reflect a calm sense of well-being, a willingness to accept the differences of others, and an orientation toward peace that makes for a stronger, more flexible, and healthier world.

Chapter 1

The Facts

Definition

Osteoporosis, or porous bone, is a disease characterized by low bone mass and structural deterioration of bone tissue, leading to bone fragility and an increased susceptibility to fractures, especially of the hip, spine, and wrist, although any bone can be affected.[1]

Epidemiology

In the hippie days of the 1960s, two fellows crossed Michigan Avenue to Chicago's Oak Street Beach. "Man, look at the water," one said. "Like, that lake is *big*." The other observed. "And that's only the top." So it is with osteoporosis. The extent of the problem is much greater than first meets the eye.

The statistics are hard to ignore: Forty-four million Americans are known to have low bone mass. That amounts to 55 percent of everyone over age 50.[2] One in two women and one in four men over age 50 will have an osteoporosis-related fracture in his or her lifetime. Osteoporosis is responsible for more than 1.5 million fractures annually, including roughly

- 300,000 hip fractures,
- 700,000 vertebral fractures,
- 250,000 wrist fractures, and
- 300,000 fractures at other sites.[3]

In 2001 more than 315,000 people were admitted to American hospitals with hip fractures, most of them due to osteoporosis.

In the year 2000 it was estimated that osteoporosis caused 37,500 deaths in the United States alone.

Men over 50 are more likely to suffer from a hip fracture than prostate cancer.[4] A woman's risk of hip fracture is equal to the combined risk of breast, uterine, and ovarian cancer.[5]

Women are as likely to die after a hip fracture as they are from breast cancer.[6]

Thirty-two percent of women will fracture a hip before reaching the age of 80. After reaching 50, the mortality rate in the first year following a hip fracture is 25 percent.[7]

Twenty percent of those who could walk before a hip fracture were relegated to long-term care afterward. The cost of hip fractures to the United States in 2002 was $18 billion.[8]

Osteoporosis is in fact a global problem, excluding no ethnic group or gender. More than 200 million people worldwide are faced with the progressive weakening of already thinned bones and the prospect of often-fatal, always painful, and disabling fractures.[9] In most cases, the medical support and financial means necessary to diagnose the condition are lacking, as are medications for its amelioration, or treatment for the fractures that will otherwise occur.

Researchers in many countries have investigated osteoporosis and contributed to its understanding. The pressure is *on* to effectively prevent and treat this threatening condition, which increases in incidence as life expectancy improves.

Why Is Osteoporosis Dangerous?

What osteoporosis does is impressively simple: It breaks bones. Spine and hip fractures grimly result in painful nights awake, invalidism, and demise.[10]

A staggering percentage of the 10 million Americans whose bones have thinned below a critical level will have spinal fractures, the most common and possibly the most painful type. Yet 34 million people have low bone strength, not quite low enough to warrant the label "osteoporosis," but significant enough to have a name of its own: *osteopenia*. Although each individual in this group has lower risk, taken as a whole, people with osteopenia will actually have more spinal fractures than people with osteoporosis.[11]

Vertebral fractures may, of course, occur as the result of a fall, but the mechanism is usually different: simple forward slumping, *kyphosis* or "dowager's hump," often seen in the later years, puts so much pressure on the forward parts of the spinal column that osteoporotic bones spontaneously collapse. This type of break is referred to as a *wedge fracture*.

The process deserves closer scrutiny. The different thoracic vertebrae are of relatively equal strength. Thoracic kyphosis places more weight on the forward part of the vertebrae. When one vertebra fractures, the angle of the spine is even more acute, and the weight of the head, shoulders, chest, arms, and vertebrae above the level of the fracture is further concentrated on the front of the spinal column. The previous angle of the uninjured spine was sufficient to cause one vertebra to collapse. The more acute angle that results from the fracture is even more likely to disrupt another vertebra. Following that event, still more angling makes a third fracture more probable. A recent article in the journal *Osteoporosis International* found that the best predictor of a vertebral fracture is a previous vertebral fracture.[12]

Hip fractures are strong and sinister, the second-most common fracture overall as well as the most lethal, with deeply felt, often lifelong or life-ending consequences.[13] Wrist, ankle, elbow, shoulder, and knee frac-

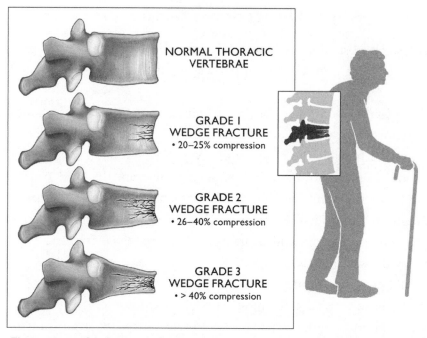

NORMAL THORACIC
VERTEBRAE

GRADE I
WEDGE FRACTURE
• 20–25% compression

GRADE 2
WEDGE FRACTURE
• 26–40% compression

GRADE 3
WEDGE FRACTURE
• > 40% compression

Figure I. *Wedge fractures often occur in a kyphotic spine. The first vertebral fracture unfortunately tends to exaggerate kyphosis still further, increasing the likelihood of a second and third fracture. Progressive grades of fracture incline the spine ever more strongly toward future injury.*

tures are also common, usually occurring when a person uses an arm or a leg to break a fall. It is the unbroken fall that fractures the hip. A new osteoporotic fracture of any kind raises the risk of mortality by 32 percent, regardless of a person's age.[14] A hip fracture subjects people to time in bed and wheelchairs, weakening muscles and bones still further, and deconditioning the balance mechanisms in the body that were already inconstant enough to produce the fracture. The fracture itself is not the killer. Mortality derives from the life changes that result: weeks of bedrest with the increased chance of pneumonia and other opportunistic infections, decubitus ulcers (bedsores), weaker muscles, digestive ills, and isolation from society, even family. It is hardly surprising that studies find loss of quality in nearly every facet of life after a hip fracture: mobility, emotional status, social interactions, and sleep, to name a few, all declined.[15]

But the seriousness of a hip fracture also stems from changes that occur before the fall that produces it. Many geriatricians feel that a hip fracture is a "sentinel event," an indication that irreversible deterioration has passed a critical point. Inevitable infirmities develop with age. As we add years, we attempt to adapt our lives to declining abilities and strength. Eventually, there is no more possibility of compensation, because all the margins of safety that our mental and physical resources can provide are, naturally, declining too. Barring a sudden event, whether we like it or not, many of us will come to a point at which we cannot adequately prepare for and protect ourselves from a fall and its unfortunate consequences. The trick, and a focus of this book, is to build bone before it weakens, countering osteoporosis as effectively and as comfortably as possible.

And like the hippie who only saw the surface of Lake Michigan, we have only scratched the surface of this topic.

Fighting osteoporosis is a lifelong battle. Like a successful general, the first thing we need is an understanding of our foe. In this chapter we'll begin with the basics of osteoporosis and how a diagnosis is made. In later chapters we'll discuss factors that influence its development, and the standard treatments. We will not be shy about finding fault with these treatments, since one needs to go into this with open eyes. It is important to bear in mind that there *is* prevention, which is always more effective than treatment, and certainly less invasive.

Diagnosis of Osteoporosis and Osteopenia

Many people assume that osteoporosis is a woman's disease. In fact, several studies show that men suffer from osteoporosis at approximately one half to one fourth the rate of women, but are diagnosed only one eighth as often.[16] In a growing and aging world population, all the osteoporosis numbers are, naturally, growing too. But men's rates are increasing faster. In New South Wales older men actually led women in ankle fractures. Also, between 1993 and 2003 the number of wrist fractures in men jumped 71 percent while women's rose 43 percent.[17] In the United States, men represent only one fifth of those diagnosed with osteoporosis, but there are one third as many osteoporotic fractures in men as in women.[18] A study in British Columbia found that in spite of the fact that only 12.5 percent of the people diagnosed with osteoporosis were men, 25 to 30 percent of all hip fractures were sustained by men.[19]

Other studies document ineffective medical intervention in the United States. One hundred and six inner-city New York women with vertebral fractures were prescribed bone density testing. Only six received it. Further, only 15 percent of the initial X-ray reports even mention the fractures.[20]

In Ann Arbor, Michigan, a telephone survey found that the only life-style adjustment 219 women made after being diagnosed with osteoporosis was to increase their use of over-the-counter calcium supplements. These patients were not impressed with the seriousness of their condition; they did not see that the disastrous future consequences of osteoporosis could threaten their well-being.[21]

This comment from another study identifies a prevalent attitude toward the disease: "Treatment of osteoporosis was more acceptable to participants than exercise classes."[22] In other words, people are inclined to wait until they have osteoporosis and then treat it, rather than being motivated to prevent it. "If it's not broken, don't fix it" unfortunately does not apply to our bones. If a bone is getting ever weaker, it needs attention now. In osteoporosis, prevention is not just the better part of cure, it's the best treatment![23]

How to Identify Osteoporosis and Follow Its Course

Since osteoporosis is a disease of bone fragility, it stands to reason that any benign test for it will measure bone strength. The gold standard today is a test for bone mineral density (BMD), which determines how thick and solid the bones are.

Every test is an abstraction. A blood test measures iron outside the context of the human body, and apart from any molecular parts to which the iron was attached; an electrocardiogram records the heart's electrical impulses without regard to its mass, bloodflow, or temperature. Similarly, we know from the outset that any measure of a bone's mass isn't going to take everything into account. In fact, the most commonly used and currently most reliable measure of its strength, bone mineral density, doesn't consider the different ways in which bones are constructed in different individuals. Moreover, the test is designed and standardized only for women.

For many years osteoporosis has turned up as an incidental finding to a chest X-ray or an X-ray of a bone following a fall. The "ground glass" or lenslike appearance of a long bone such as the femur or humerus is often the tip-off. But the definitive test for osteoporosis is the dual-energy X-ray absorptiometry (DEXA) scan. This X-ray involves so little radiation that the radiology technicians administering it do not wear lead aprons, though they conduct the tests every day. Nevertheless, it is an extremely valuable guide to whether a patient has osteoporosis and whether efforts to counter its progression are effective.

What Is a DEXA Scan?

Osteoporosis, weakening of the bones, is not exactly uniform; some bones may be weaker than others. It is, however, largely a systemic process, affecting all the bones. Modern medical science has defined osteoporosis as a significantly abnormal finding in a specific examination, the DEXA scan. Bone mineral density is measured by determining the amount of energy that is absorbed as X-rays penetrate particular bones. This is proportional to the amount of calcium and other minerals that a particular cross-section of the bone contains: the more minerals, the more X-rays get absorbed. Most DEXA scans study the lumbar vertebral bodies, the iliac bone in the pelvis, and the femur, since those are the bones most commonly fractured.

The DEXA scan's reading tells how much mineral material stands between the device emitting the X-rays and the collecting plate. Two factors affect the measurement: how densely packed the bone is, and its physical dimensions. A thinner but more closely packed bone might end up with the same reading as a physically larger but less dense one. The reading is only a measure of the quantity of mineral in the tissue X-rayed.

Of course, bone mineral density is not the only factor that determines how likely a person is to have a fracture. The length of one's bones, whether they are well or poorly knit together, and how many internal cross-struts prop them up are all contributors, as are one's balance, mental status, and customary walking surface. But in spite of our ignorance about a bone's inner construction, and even discounting personal and environmental factors, we know that the lower the bone mineral density on the DEXA scan, the higher the risk of fracture.[24] In a one-year study of 197,848 postmenopausal American women of five ethnicities, a decrease of one standard deviation in BMD was matched by a 50 percent increased fracture risk in each ethnic group.[25] But what is a standard deviation?

In order to understand the result of your DEXA scan, you'll need to know a bit about statistics. Your measurement is going to be compared to that of others, specifically the "average" measurement of people at the peak of their bone strength, and people of your own age and height.

The *standard deviation*, also referred to by the Greek letter sigma, σ, is a numerical measure of how tightly the members of a group cluster together. It tells you how far different individuals in a group stray from the group's average, or *mean*. The mathematical formula determines exactly how far away from the average different proportions of the group can be found. If you look at a "normal" distribution, 68.2 percent of the group will always be located within exactly one standard deviation above and below the mean. A larger standard deviation means that the group is spread out, and 68.2 percent of the group will still be one standard deviation or less away from the mean, but that distance will be farther away from the mean, because the standard deviation is bigger. There is, of course, an average value in any case, but with a larger standard deviation many individuals will differ quite substantially from that average. A smaller standard deviation indicates that most of the group is close to the average.

The standard deviation will vary according to the discrepancy between the average value and the different individual values, but it will always include 68.2 percent of the values. Two standard deviations will include 95 percent of the values. And only 1 percent of the group will lie farther than two and a half standard deviations beyond the mean.

Using this calculation, medical researchers can determine how significantly different from the average a given value is, and what the odds are that this value represents a truly abnormal condition, rather than one that might occur just by chance.

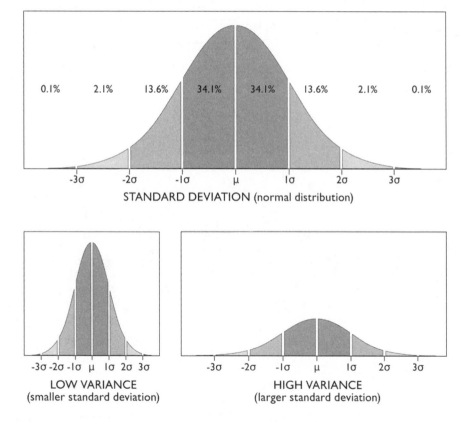

Figure 2. *In each case the standard deviation (σ) marks out the distance from the mean (μ) that includes 68.2 percent of the values.*

An Example: How Standard Deviations Work

Suppose a group of children had nothing better to do than shoot arrows, trying to land them in the bull's-eye of a large, reasonably distant target. Suppose further that by dusk there were one thousand arrows arrayed on all sides of the target. Two possible outcomes are shown in figure 3.

If we wanted to know how close the average arrow came, we could do it by measuring each arrow's distance from the bull's-eye, adding them all up, and dividing by the total number of arrows: suppose one arrow in figure 3A was 4 feet from the bull's-eye, another 14 feet, another 9 feet, another 23 feet, and so on, and that if you added up all the distances, the number for the 1,000 arrows came to 10,000. The average distance that arrows lay from the bull's-eye would therefore be 10 feet. Calculating the standard deviation tells you how diverse the positions of the different arrows are, based on how far they array themselves from 10, the mean. Statisticians use a formula that goes through each arrow's distance, sub-

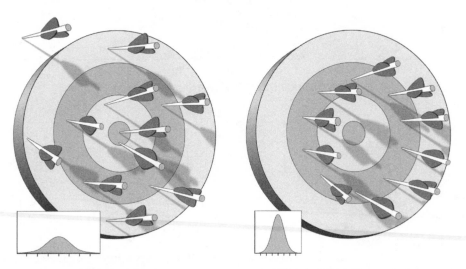

A. HIGH VARIANCE (larger standard deviation)   B. LOW VARIANCE (smaller standard deviation)

Figure 3. *Even though both sets of arrows have the same average distance from the bull's-eye, their standard deviations are very different.*

tracting it from 10, and squaring it. The greater the resulting number, the higher the standard deviation. As anyone can see, these arrows' positions are quite diverse, so the number will be big.

Now examine the second picture, figure 3B, and consider the standard deviation. Once again the average distance of any arrow from the bull's-eye is 10 feet. But the standard deviation, determined by subtracting each individual arrow's distance from the average distance, will be very small. That small number reflects the fact that the arrows' distance from the bull's eye are nearly identical.

In the first picture, an arrow that's 20 feet from the center is nothing remarkable. Even though it's twice the average distance, that sort of thing happened frequently. Another way of saying this is that the standard deviation is very large. An arrow that lands 20 feet from the bull's-eye is, therefore, less than one standard deviation beyond the mean, and a fairly probable event.

We see clusters of things all the time, from the size of people's footprints at the beach to scores on national tests. A very tight clustering of values is remarkable, and makes us ask "What would make the arrows line up as they did in figure 3B?" Possibly tornado-like winds, or a magnetic vortex that gripped every arrow-tip and whirled it down in a tight ring. We do not know why, but the power of statistics is such that we do not need to. Given the standard deviation of the situation depicted in figure 3B, an arrow falling 20 feet beyond the bull's-eye would be a most unlikely thing. This position would be many standard deviations beyond the mean. It would require an explanation.

Your Diagnosis

The standard DEXA test in the United States scans three sites: the lumbar vertebrae, the total hip, and the surgical neck of the thigh bone. The image your bones generate in the DEXA scan is compared with the average image seen in healthy 25- to 30-year-old women, and with average healthy women of your age, height, and weight. Your T-score is how many standard deviations your measured bone mineral density is beyond the average DEXA value seen in healthy women between 25 and 30 years of age; the Z-score is how many standard deviations your score lies beyond the average DEXA value seen in healthy women of your age, height, and weight. A positive score puts you above the average, a negative score indicates that the average person has stronger bones than you do. If your T-score falls 2.5 standard deviations below the mean, indicating that your bones are weaker than 99 percent of women between ages 25 and 30, women at the peak of their bone strength, then you've got osteoporosis. T-scores that fall between 1.0 and 2.5 standard deviations below the mean indicate osteopenia, a danger zone—the bones are approaching an osteoporotic state. The DEXA-based diagnostic criteria are quite precise. If the T-score at any of the three sites reaches either of these values, then the diagnosis is made.

How Reliable Is the DEXA Scan?

The correlation between a low bone mineral density reading on the DEXA scan and a fracture is stronger than the relationship between high blood pressure and stroke.[26] Still, the test is not universally or entirely accurate. DEXA scans detect 9 out of 10 people with osteoporosis and

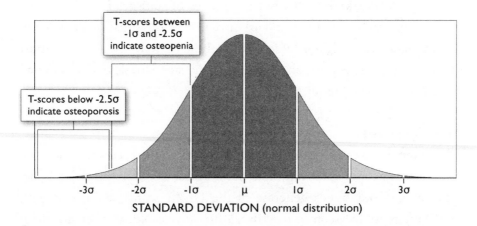

Figure 4. *T-scores lower than approximately two thirds of young women indicate osteopenia. T-scores below 99 percent of young women indicate osteoporosis.*

wrongly diagnose healthy people somewhere between 5 and 7 percent of the time.

There is a 3–4 percent margin of error in the instruments.[27] if your score has fallen no more than 0.1, don't take it too seriously, since a number of external conditions may affect the accuracy of the test. These include

- Spinal surgery,
- Hardware (certain pain-relief devices, or plates, rods, or screws used to fix broken bones),
- Vertebral deformities, including arthritis and previous fractures, and
- Calcified blood vessels that may lie close to the spinal column.

Women should not undergo DEXA scans during pregnancy. Even the minuscule amounts of radiation emitted by the bone scan are thought harmful to a fetus. For patients with any conditions that contraindicate a DEXA scan, there are other tests. The peripheral dual-energy X-ray absorptiometry (pDEXA) measures bone density in distal bones, such as the finger, wrist, and heel. Single-energy X-ray absorptiometry (SEXA) uses a small, portable device similar to the DEXA scanner, but it emits a single X-ray beam rather than two. It is used to measure bone density in the heel or forearm. If results are abnormal, and a more specific test such as the standard DEXA scan cannot be performed, it is wisest to treat the individual just as one would if the DEXA scan were positive.[28]

There are other ways to diagnose osteoporosis and osteopenia. Ultrasound, particularly of the heel or the wrist bones, is used when the DEXA scan is either unavailable or inadvisable.[29] Magnetic resonance imaging (MRI) and computed tomography (CT) scanning are used today in research, such as bone quality studies. They are also valuable under special conditions when other diagnostic possibilities loom, such as the bone-affecting cancer multiple myeloma, or metabolic or nutritional states such as osteomalacia.

Whether detected through DEXA, pDEXA, SEXA, ultrasound, MRI, or CT scanning, the idea is always the same: Thin and weak bones are vulnerable to fracture. How vulnerable?

Bone Density and Fracture Risk

One standard deviation below the mean in a T-score comes out somewhere between 2.0 and 2.6 times greater probability of hip fracture. The correlation between BMD and fracture risk is so strong that researchers at Washington University have constructed a "fracture risk calculator" to estimate fracture risk based on bone density; you can try it yourself at http://courses.washington.edu/bonephys/FxRiskCalculator.html.

Yet we must bear in mind that the risk of fracture in any given individual is a function of other factors as well:

1. Gender and age (see figure 5)
2. Bone quality: This subject is being pursued quite vigorously today. New micro-MRI technology and fractal analysis may enable research that assesses the importance of bones' inner structure in their ability to resist fracture.
3. Sensory losses: Any deficit of sight, hearing, or the ability to feel one's feet increases the danger of a fall. Those in need should be encouraged to use eyeglasses, hearing aids, and assistive devices. This is especially true for people with osteoporosis.
4. Activity level: More daily activity will strengthen bones, but higher activity levels also put people at greater risk. Pick your exercise carefully.

As with just about any medical condition, there are two sides to fracture: *susceptibility*, that is, bone fragility, and *exposure*, that is, the history and environment that determines your risk of falling. Race-car drivers have a higher risk of fracture, regardless of their DEXA scores.

One reliable measure of susceptibility and exposure to falls, the Morse Fall Scale, sums mental status, independence in walking, any other diagnoses, IV or heparin-lock use, and, naturally, any history of falls. On this basis

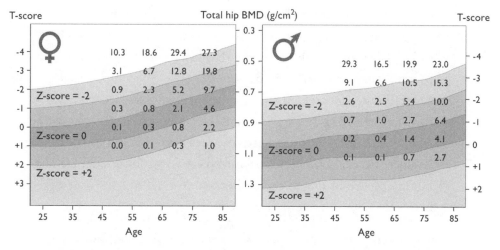

Figure 5. *The relationship between bone density and factor risk is shown in results from a 39,000-patient study conducted in Europe, North America, and Japan.* [30]

the scale determines your risk of sustaining a fracture, very much like the way college admission committees determine whether candidates will make the grade.[31] The Cummings Hip Scale uses physical and social function, bodily pain, emotional role, mental health, and general vigor to calculate the same thing.[32] Both methods quantify an individual's exposure to falls, and therefore an appropriate level of concern about having strong bones.

Your Allies against Fractures

Fractures from falls are so detrimental to health that it is important to marshal all forces against them. Exposure to risk can be reduced, but the aging processes are inexorable. It makes sense to initiate contrary processes that are stronger. There are three basic elements to work on:

- Strength. Greater muscular strength puts greater strain on the bones in almost every action. The stress stimulates the bones to create more bone tissue. Greater strength also better counters gravity, reducing vulnerability to falling. Be aware that muscular strength can overpower bone strength. We once treated a circus strong man who had met a strong man from another circus. Unsurprisingly, they arm wrestled. His humerus was broken in three places: the combined strength of their biceps (and their wills to win) were stronger than his bone!

- Mental status. Decreased ability to recognize objects, such as furniture, automobiles, and staircases; reduced alertness; and confusion lead to fracturing falls. Less activity goes with lower mental status.
- Balance. People with better balance have fewer falls. A simple fact, but an important one to remember.

Naturally these are interrelated: a person of low activity level is, insofar as that is concerned, at lower risk of fracture. But strength, balance, and bone quality (as well as bone density) all tend to improve with greater activity. On the other hand, for a person of lower mental status, a person who is disoriented, extremely forgetful, or distractible, higher activity is definitely a higher risk. It is important to choose the right level of activity for an individual's condition.

Chapter 2

Bones

What is a bone?

The tissue comprising bone has two components: a protein matrix or *osteoid*, which is produced by *osteocytes*, and the mineral elements that become lodged within it. The mineral elements are chiefly calcium and

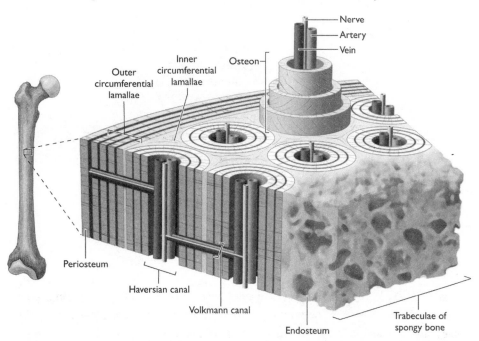

Figure 6. *Bones are an intricate latticework of live cells, the channels that feed and interrelate them, their proteinaceous secretions, and the minerals the proteins draw into their structure.* After L. C. Junqueira and J. Carniero, *Basic Histology*, 10th ed. (New York: McGraw-Hill, 2003), p. 144.

phosphate. There are smaller amounts of bicarbonate, citrate, potassium, sodium, and magnesium. Each element is replaced periodically.

The minerals calcium and phosphate form a crystal-like structure, *hydroxyapatite*, with chemical formula $Ca_{10}(PO_4)_6(OH)_2$.

Both protein and mineral elements are necessary for bones to have their essential characteristics. We can understand the function of these elements by observing what happens when they are missing. In *osteomalacia*, a disease in which bones do not have enough calcium, the bones are soft and bending, not supportive. When the protein elements are removed experimentally from normal bones, they crumble like chalk.

There are a number of subtle balances here, too. Even the metabolic process has a requisite speed. Protein's life cycle has its own timing, like the tempering of steel. When the process is hurried, problems occur, as in an unusual medical condition, osteitis fibrosa cystica, which results in

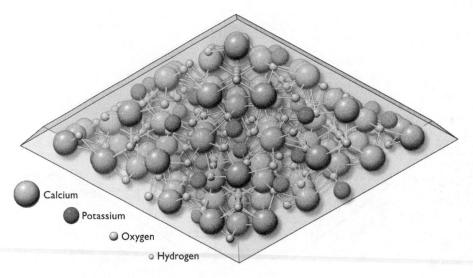

Calcium
Potassium
Oxygen
Hydrogen

Figure 7. *The hydroxyapatite crystals function in bone just as metal reinforcement bars do in concrete. A coating of water surrounding the crystals of calcium and phosphate enables them to pass in and out of the bloodstream.* After M. I. Kay, R. A. Young, and A. S. Pesner, "Crystal Structure of Hydroxyapatite," *Nature* 204 (December 1964): 1050–1052, used with permission of Sigma=Aldrich Company, St. Louis, Missouri.

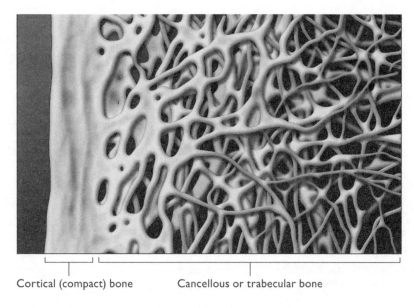

Cortical (compact) bone   Cancellous or trabecular bone

Figure 8. *Compact or cortical bone and cancellous or trabecular bone.* Adapted from Junqueira and Carniero, p. 145, with permission of the publisher.

fibrous bones. Failure of a child's bones to pick up adequate minerals from the available dietary sources or from the bloodstream results in rickets, bones that bend under the strains of daily life.

As already mentioned, adults who are losing boney mineral have osteomalacia, too little calcium per volume of bone. But too much calcium, which results in the condition *osteopetrosis*, isn't good either—the marrow cavities where blood cells are made become narrow and are eventually obliterated, leading to anemia that may be fatal.

Too little protein and inadequate mineral content have effects similar to osteoporosis: the chances of fracture increase. But neither condition is the same as osteoporosis, where the proportions of protein and mineral in the bone are well-balanced, there are just less of them. But there is more to the story of bones than their composition. Another important contrast highlights a critical characteristic of almost every bone.

The Structure of Bone

We know that osteoid and minerals make up the basic substance of bone, but what form do these elements take? We know *what* bones are made of, but *how* are they constructed? Bones actually have two distinct parts. The compact part, the *cortex* or *cortical bone*, forms a hard shell just below the surface. The spongy part, the *cancellous* or *trabecular bone*, lies deeper within. The strength of each varies along with the proportions of its two main components, the protein spicules that make up the matrix, and the calcium and other minerals that are attracted to the matrix and harden it. Both are composed of the same osteoid matrix and hydroxyapatite core, but they are different.

Cortical bone forms a hard outer ring and constitutes a large part of any bone's strength. While there are variations in the mineral content of cortical bone, it is more or less the same thickness, and has essentially the same form in just about everyone.

Although there are certainly variations in the consistency and strength of cortical bone, by far the greater variations appear to be within the trabecular region, with its variably formed and differently angled inner struts and latticework. Bone density is responsible for only 60 percent of bone strength and consequent likelihood of fracture. The other 40 percent appears to be due to the formations of the trabecular bone.[1]

The strength of this structural formation may be calculated by a formula developed by the great Swiss mathematician Leonhard Euler (1707–1783). Euler's buckling theory states that the strength of a vertically compressed strut is inversely proportional to the square of the unsupported length, that is, the distance between its transverse struts.[2]

Both the mineral content and the geometric conformation of the elements contribute to what is known as bone quality. Quality enters into any logical assessment of bone strength: Two bones of the same density may be structured differently. You don't need a degree from MIT to know that the George Washington Bridge can support more weight than a helter-skelter pile of the same materials.

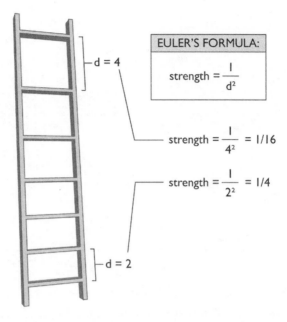

EULER'S FORMULA:

$$\text{strength} = \frac{1}{d^2}$$

$$\text{strength} = \frac{1}{4^2} = 1/16$$

$$\text{strength} = \frac{1}{2^2} = 1/4$$

Figure 9. *Two parallel columns with struts 4 inches apart at the top, and two inches apart on the bottom. The parallel columns will support four times more weight at the bottom.*

At this writing, what determines a bone's structure, and what might change it, are not precisely known. But a good deal of research is focused on finding the answer. Certain genetic, environmental, hormonal, drug-related, and dietary influences are already known,[3] but any notions of the precise ways to influence bone quality are largely hypotheses in the minds of scientists, physicians, and yogis.

The fracture risk inherent in bone is determined by two physical factors: bone density and bone quality. Bone density is well understood and can be accurately measured. Bone quality is currently under intense investigation. Considerations such as mental status, activity level, and environmental factors—stairs and rugs in the home, slippery surfaces, and occupation—are all relevant, but currently, all other things being equal, the most reliable test we have for the risk of fractures is still the DEXA scan for bone mineral density.

Until recently, the only way to assess overall bone quality was to take

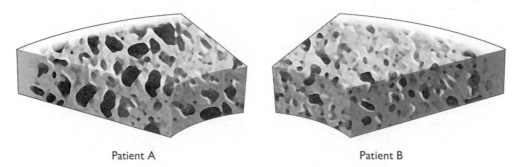

Patient A   Patient B

Figure 10. *Two patients' bones with the same DEXA score but possibly quite different strength.*

a biopsy. The high cost of a biopsy and its invasive nature discouraged its use in the general population. But a virtual bone biopsy, a noninvasive tool for bone quality assessment, is already being tested. Micro-MRI studies find striking differences between different individual's bones, and these differences are almost sure to relate to the bones' strength.[4]

The virtual bone biopsy may be an important tool in monitoring patient treatment. Figure 10 shows the structural images of bones from two women who have similar DEXA T-scores, yet quite different trabecular bone structure. The current standard practice would have both women receive the same treatment. However, the structural characteristics of the bones, determined by the virtual assay and computed along the lines of Euler's formula, suggest that Patient A may be at a significantly higher risk for fractures. If that is the case, then the nature and intensity of the treatment of these two patients should be adjusted accordingly. If both patients are receiving the same treatment, we may speculate that Patient A is not receiving the aggressive treatment she truly needs. Patient B may be suffering needlessly from the side effects of medications she doesn't require.

How Bones Grow

Bones begin to develop long before an infant leaves the womb, lengthening until approximately age 17, and strengthening until age 25 or 30.

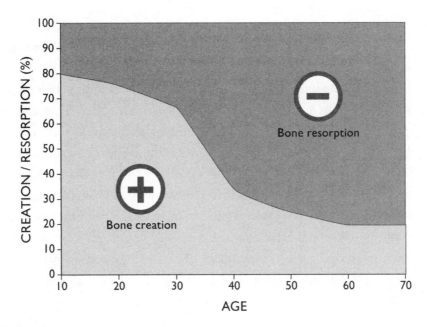

Figure 11. *On average, a woman's bones stop getting stronger and start weakening quite dramatically between age 30 and 40.* Adapted from G. Kessler, *The Bone Density Program* (New York: Ballantine Books, 2001), p. 393.

Although the length of bones does not change significantly after age 30, their strength declines as hormones change in midlife; that decline tapers off after age 65.[5] While bone loss actually slows down after 65, this inexorable cumulative bone loss is responsible for most osteoporosis.

All bones, long or short, round or flat, men's or women's, are constantly subject to two processes: one builds up their mass and strength, and one eats their substance away. Like just about every tissue in the body, and the quiet imperishable quality of life itself, there is an incessant metabolism, a constant flux of the constituents of bone.

There are the osteoblasts, which are themselves derived from cartilage-making cells, the chondrocytes. These cells secrete collagen, proteoglycans, and glycoproteins that form a woven organic fabric of proteins, the aforementioned osteoid. The matrix then attracts calcium and phosphates to make up the molecule hydroxyapatite (see figure 7). Some of the flat bones spring directly from osteoblasts' secretions; other bones, the long bones of the arms and legs, first appear in small cartilaginous forms that subsequently ossify.

The osteoblasts form a thin lining around the bones until they incorporate themselves into it. At that point they become osteocytes. They change shape, from rectangular to star-shaped, with long thin tendrils that connect to other osteocytes. Ultimately, the first ones in these lines of connected cells link up to a blood vessel—one of the tiny capillaries—for exchange of nutrients and the products of metabolism. It is believed that a chain of as many as 15 osteocytes can effectively transport substances to and from the one that's farthest from the central canal containing a blood vessel and a nerve.

The metamorphoses of osteoblasts, the cells they come from (chondrocytes), and the cells they may become (osteocytes) are all sensitive to

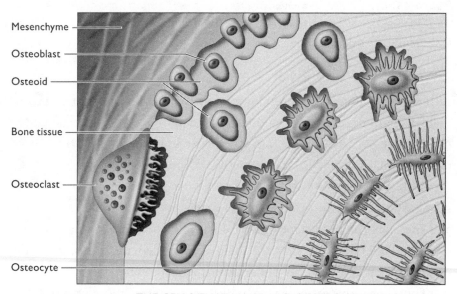

THE CELLS THAT MAKE AND DESTROY BONE

Figure 12. *Ovoid osteoblasts turn into the star-shaped osteocytes as they surround themselves with the protein they synthesize. The process is complete when minerals are attracted to their secretion, turning it into bone, within which the osteocytes soon find themselves deeply embedded. Osteoclasts reabsorb diseased and dying fragments of bone.* After Junqueira and Carniero, p. 142, with permission of the publisher.

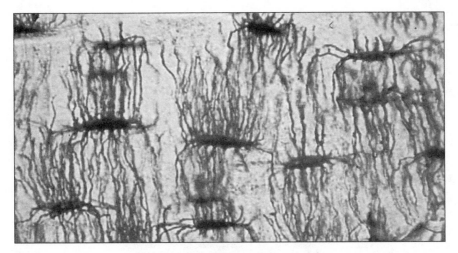

OSTEOCYTES IN COMMUNICATION

Figure 13. *Nutrients and chemical "messages" are telegraphed through as many as 15 osteocytes that are otherwise alienated from the rest of the body by the density of their own secretions.* From Junqueira and Carniero, p. 141, with permission of the publisher.

a number of hormonal influences—progesterone, estrogen, testosterone, growth hormone, thyroid hormones, and parathyroid hormone all play a role. We will come to them soon. This controlled conversion has one more relevant participant, *osteoclasts*, which are responsible for a different, antagonistic process.

Osteoclasts are strange and gigantic cells, derived from bone marrow, that can often have more than 50 nuclei. They literally digest bone, sending the protein and minerals they swallow back into the bloodstream. They are attracted to injured and old sections of bone and to places where the supporting osteocytes have died, leaving a region of bone unattended. Not unlike a moray eel, they fasten themselves tightly to the affected bone through their "ruffled zone," a tightly walled-off space into which they send collagenase, other digestive enzymes, and acidic components. This caustic cocktail decomposes the bone. After absorption into the osteoclast, the protein is digested further, and then its components, along with the minerals, are released back into the body's general circulation.

Many factors affect the behavior of osteoclasts. Some are relatively

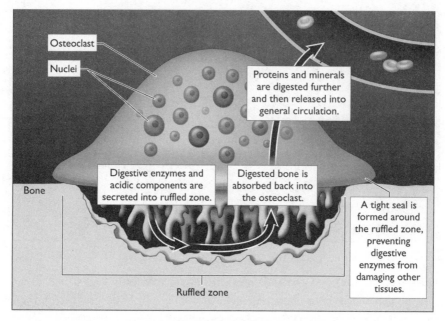

AN OSTEOCLAST AT WORK

Figure 14. *Many nuclei are found in one osteoclast, probably because so many diverse tasks must be completed to undo the body's work of crafting bone. These complex cells can undo a skeleton that could otherwise endure thousands of years of wind and weather.* From Junqueira and Carniero, p. 143, with permission of the publisher.

simple. Osteoclasts are inhibited by calcitonin, a hormone secreted by the thyroid gland. Parathyroid hormone, on the other hand, has contradictory effects: this hormone stimulates osteocytes, the osteoclasts' competitor, activating them so that they produce more protein and secrete a molecule that arouses the osteoclasts. Therefore, a parathyroid hormone directly stimulates the -blasts and indirectly stimulates the -clasts, an intercellular system of checks and balances.

Balance: The Elusive Key

What governs the all-important rates of the two processes of bone creation and resorption? There are a number of factors that are not fully understood. We do know enough, however, to appreciate the complexity of the relationship and to explore some ways to manipulate the processes in our bones' favor. For example, at low blood serum levels, parathyroid hormone stimulates bone-building osteocytes, but at higher concentrations it reduces the mineral content of the forearm bones.[6] Phosphorus gets into the act as well, but too much phosphate will change the absorption of calcium. This in turn will alter parathyroid hormone levels, which will then feed back to change absorption yet again.

These seemingly opposed biologic processes cooperate beautifully under normal circumstances. Atomic force microscopic studies, finer than electron microscopy for these purposes, have seen osteoclasts munching away at corners of bone where microcracks have appeared. This suggests that at the "local level" osteoclasts are drawn to these defects (by a process we do not presently understand) and begin to create excavation sites at which bone resorption is taking place. The calcium thus reclaimed is free for the osteocytes to pick out of the bloodstream to re-create healthy bone at spots where it had been damaged.[7]

Research has uncovered this critical aspect of inborn maintenance capacity: When osteocytes die, the adjacent bone regions are no longer supported, and the tissue becomes resorbed by the osteoclasts. There are definite chemical signals for this clean-up operation, and different factors maintain the status quo, keeping osteoclastic activity at bay. Balancing and regulating these processes is the principal way in which many of the anti-osteoporosis drugs work. One must be aware of these checks and balances and some of their advantages to appreciate the rewards and risks of using the drugs. Before considering the treatment, though, it makes sense to look at the disease: What makes bones brittle in the first place?

Chapter 3

Factors That Affect Bones

What makes or breaks a bone?

God grant me the serenity
to accept the things I cannot change;
courage to change the things I can;
and wisdom to know the difference.

—REINHOLD NIEBUHR, 1892–1971

It is important to have some understanding of the factors that contribute to bone formation, regardless of whether one has any conscious control over them. Age, genetics, hormones, and nutrition all influence bone formation, as well as the disintegration that leads to osteopenia and osteoporosis. Information about how these factors come into play is valuable for younger people, to prevent bone weakening, and for older individuals, to recover bone density. Young or old, we should all feel respect, even awe, for the complex, sensitive, yet robust organisms we are.

Age

Age is an obvious, reliable factor that determines one's risk for fracture. In a study of 200,160 women, researchers at Columbia University came up with results that fit neatly in a small table.

Age	Risk of Fracture
50–64	31%
65+	62%

They corroborated the findings from another large study in which each standard deviation below the mean value of bone mineral density increased the risk of fracture 50 percent.[1]

No one can entirely halt the aging process, but we can control lifestyle, which can affect bone density and can increase or decrease your risk of fracture in as little as two years.

Perhaps the most important thing about age is how to take advantage of it. We all build up the most bone we'll ever have by age 30. After that the bones tend to thin and weaken. So the very best thing we can do is generate a high peak bone mass before age 30. It's best to combat osteoporosis when you are young and do not have it.

There is an accelerating rate of bone loss after age 30 (see figure 11 in chapter 2). If you build up your bones while you're young, then it will take longer for the predictable drop in bone mass to cross the –2.5 T-score line. This type of prevention is not new. By the same rationale children are given inoculations for diphtheria, whooping cough, and tetanus before they've ever gone to school or stepped on a rusty nail. It's why smoking is never a good idea (for your bones or your lungs). Osteoporosis is best countered through prevention.

Anti-osteoporosis exercises should be taught in gym class in schools. Volleyball is a dandy game, and works to build bones, but few play it after the age of 50, when slowing down the bone thinning process is so critical. And does volleyball take your peak mineral density over the top as the ball sails over the net? Who knows? Yoga is probably the best and most long-lived lesson that gym teachers could impart to their students. Yoga builds muscle strength and joint flexibility and improves balance and posture, all while promoting calm, considered response to life's challenges. This whole book is an argument for precisely this teaching!

Genetics

Some studies find that ethnic groups have different boney characteristics: An American study of 197,848 people recorded BMD and fracture in women from five ethnic groups: 7,784 African Americans, 1,912 Asians, 6,973 Latin Americans, 1,708 Native Americans, and 179,471 whites, none of whose boney strengths were known at the start.[2] By the time they reached the age of 80, more than 20 percent of the women in each ethnic group had bone mineral density T-scores below –2.5. They had osteoporosis. African American women had the highest BMD; Asian women had the lowest. One year after the study began, 2,414 new fractures of the spine, hip, forearm, wrist, or rib appeared. White and Latin American women had the highest risk for fracture, Native Americans were next, then African Americans, and last Asian Americans.

There *is* a correlation between BMD and likelihood of fracture: The lower the T-scores, the greater the risk of fracture within each group. But obviously there are other factors at work here, since overall Asian Americans had the lowest BMD, but also the lowest risk of fracture. Heredity probably plays a role in bone development.

Heredity is probably not, however, a primary factor. In one study, hereditary factors were estimated for 3,320 people in southern China. Researchers studied environmental differences, such as calcium intake, smoking status, phytoestrogen intake, exercise, and alcohol consumption. The environmental factors altered the heritable BMD, but did so differently in males and females. Females were found to be more sensitive to environmental changes than men, and therefore were better able to alter their BMD through diet and exercise.[3]

BMD increases in immigrants to the United States from Africa in direct proportion to their length of residence, another example of the power of factors such as nutrition, activity, and general well-being.[4]

Hormones

Manipulating hormone levels is beyond the scope and purpose of this book, but a clear acquaintance with their positive and negative influence is an advantage. Understanding the complexities of what we can and cannot alter is always good.

Hormones present a situation in which we definitely have some control, but it is limited. Most hormones can be created synthetically, and overactive glands can be removed surgically. There are homeostatic and feedback loops that provide for a good deal of self-adjustment. Nevertheless, the balance, the equilibrium points, the greater harmonies of the entire orchestra do not always come naturally. If they did, there would be no need for the medications or the surgeries.

Bone tissue is quite sensitive to hormonal changes. Estrogen, testosterone, growth hormone, parathyroid hormone, calcitonin, and thyroid hormone all have positive and negative effects on the processes that maintain strong and healthy bones. Naturally, there are genetic factors that influence hormonal timing and balance. But contemporary medicine can monitor all the hormones and therefore their balance. Further, the surgical, chemical, radioactive, and nutritionally supplementary alterations can be monitored too.

Estrogen and Testosterone

Estrogen generally seems to affect the dual processes of laying down and reabsorbing the cancellous/trabecular bone. In a well-controlled German study on rats, estrogen and testosterone seemed to play a part in improving the trabecular region's density. Estrogen improved mechanical stability; testosterone did not.[5]

In another rat study, British researchers found just the opposite mechanism: Bone-making cells, the osteocytes, responded positively to both strain and estrogen. Ninety percent of the effect was seen in the compact, or cortical, bone. This study is one of many that link estrogen to bones' response to strain. Estrogen seems to enhance the body's bone-making capacity following pressure. This is the reason exercise in the first few decades of life when estrogen levels are highest is so vital to successfully resisting osteoporosis.[6]

Testosterone seems to have even more of an effect. An Estonian study of sixty boys between ages 10 and 18 found that testosterone levels were the best predictor of hip, lower spine, and pelvic bone mineral density.[7]

We can conclude that the effect of exercise will be amplified or minimized depending upon the amount of estrogen or estrogen-like substances in the blood. Testosterone exerts perhaps an even stronger influence in building healthy bone mass. It can be hypothesized that bones build up before age 30 because estrogen and testosterone production is highest at that time.

Growth Hormone

The Estonian study also found that relative amounts of free insulin-like growth factor (IGF) are strongly correlated with bone mineral density.[8] IGF, a hormone-like protein, comes in two forms. IGF-1 is active in almost every adult cell and is secreted by the liver. IGF-2 is critical for early development of the brain and bones of the fetus, and is secreted by the brain, kidneys, muscles, and pancreas. Exercise seems to stimulate their secretion.

It will not come as a surprise that growth hormone influences bone growth in children. It is also well known that excessive growth hormone in later years produces acromegaly, a condition in which the long bones get thicker, but neither longer nor stronger. It is unclear whether this condition artificially elevates the T- and Z-scores of a DEXA scan.

Parathyroid Hormone

Parathyroid hormone (PTH) has very complex and important effects on bone. It is a leading cause of osteopenia, and yet paradoxically it also helps build new bone.[9] One European study suggests that within reasonable limits, the full parathyroid hormone molecule stimulates bone resorption, while one of the naturally occurring fragments of the molecule increases bone production. The study goes on to report that the ratio of these two molecular pieces in the bloodstream is influenced by heritable characteristics, underlying kidney ailments, vitamin D levels, corticosteroids, and phosphate-related factors.[10] One of these molecular fragments might lurk behind the dual mechanism whereby the parathyroid hormone acts directly on osteocytes, causing them to start producing bone, and simultaneously stimulates them to begin secreting a factor that activates osteoclasts, promoting bone loss.

To complicate things further, estrogen deficiency seems to increase the bones' receptivity to PTH, which induces them to give up more calcium to the bloodstream. The higher blood calcium serves to decrease the parathyroid glands' PTH secretion, decrease vitamin D production, and slow calcium absorption from the intestines. Poor absorption especially weakens trabecular bone, opening the door to vertebral and wrist fractures. Independent research has shown that parathyroid abnormalities are also associated with osteoporosis in the forearm bones.[11]

Calcitonin

The second of the thyroid gland's hormone trio that helps regulate mineral metabolism, calcitonin, responds to high calcium and phosphorus levels. Its primary effects are to reduce osteoclastic resorption of calcium and increase its urinary excretion, thereby lowering the blood calcium, a critical task in humans and most mammals. It does not have a very strong effect, and although it might seem like a paradox, this is highly desirable.

Our normal calcium levels have a very narrow range of safe fluctuation. Just a little too high and calcium will be deposited in our organs and other tissues, with disastrous results. But if the level falls very much, muscles go into deep and possibly fatal spasm. Remember, the heart is a muscle. Since tight control of calcium levels is critical to life, a redundant system has developed over the millennia. Since it can safely vary so little, a weak adjuster, one that responds to overabundance quickly but has a meek effect, is the perfect fine-tuner.

Nevertheless, calcitonin, a 32 amino-acid protein that is found throughout backbone-supported members of the animal kingdom, can be used as a medicine for people with too much calcium in their blood, and is effective against certain types of osteoporosis in pharmacological doses that are significantly greater than what the body produces on its own (see chapter 4).

Thyroid Hormone

Thyroxin encourages metabolism of just about every kind. Hyperthyroidism means accelerated heart rate, raised body temperature, and big appetite but thin body, all due to the increased rate of energy production and use. Hypothyroidism implies just the reverse. The person with the normal thyroid appears to have the best bones.

To state what is probably obvious: Bone growth and health are strongly influenced by hormones. The physiology and interrelationships of hormones require individual medical consultation. Being alert to the effects of hormones helps one to know when medical advice should be sought.

Nutrition

When it comes to eating and strong bones, there are do's and don'ts.

Do's

A wealth of nutrition research supports the idea of a diet high in protein and calcium, up to five servings of vegetables daily (particularly brightly colored ones), and adequate sunshine or vitamin D supplementation during early growth and the teen years. Several studies provide substantial evidence that a combination of calcium and regular exercise improves the bone mineral density in girls between the ages of 16 and 18.[12]

While finding things to eat is straightforward, understanding how nutrients work is certainly not. For example, vitamin D behaves similarly to some hormones and alters their efficiency and function. In 2002, the Women's Health Initiative conducted a randomized, controlled study of 36,202 postmenopausal women. One group of women took 1,000 mg of calcium and 400 international units of vitamin D daily for seven years; the other did not. The calcium group's bone density at the hip rose 1.06 percent, and that small increase meant that the risk of hip fracture plummeted to 71 percent of the control group's. Unfortunately, there was a significant increase in kidney stones (approximately 17 percent in those who received the calcium and vitamin D).[13] A recent study in New Zealand linked previously considered "reasonable" amounts of calcium to a significantly, increased risk of heart attack and stroke.[14] Other studies have suggested similar results.[15]

Calcium. Several experts in the field have formulated basic guidelines for calcium intake. If you are over age 75, or have problems with circulation involving either your heart or your brain, then restrict yourself to 500 mg of calcium each day. Otherwise, 1,000 to 1,500 mg per day appears to be fine.

In the healthy person under age 75, a daily dose of 1,200 to 1,500 mg of calcium is optimal. That might mean a glass of milk (300 mg), a cup of yogurt (close to 500 mg), a serving of cheese (100–300 mg), or a dish that includes dairy, such as an enchilada, lasagna, or quiche (300 mg). Among nondairy foods, fish (100–300 mg), tofu processed with calcium chloride (400 mg), soy beans and collard greens (200–350 mg), nori and sesame seeds, fortified grapefruit and orange juice (300 mg), and even mineral water (200 mg) are high scorers. Be aware that while many dairy products are fortified with calcium and vitamin D, cheese is made from milk that is not. Also, bear in mind that the USDA recommends 800 mg of calcium per day; we're advocating at least 1,200 mg, so labeling may be misleading. Unless you are wildly overfed calcium, don't worry, your body will absorb what it needs and pass on the rest.

Dr. George Kessler has written an excellent, practical book, *The Bone Density Program*, that focuses on nutrition. But as Kessler points out, all the calcium in the world won't do you any good without vitamin D or its active derivatives.

Vitamin D. The hormone-like derivatives of vitamin D are organically converted from vitamin D in sun-exposed skin. Once activated, they promote calcium and phosphorus absorption and hold the parathyroid ratios in line. They are produced only during exposure to the sun.[16] The minimum daily requirement of 20 minutes of sunshine per day can be sidestepped only by taking artificially synthesized forms of the active version, vitamin D_3. If you take the synthesized versions (as you must if you are confined indoors), they'll do the job. The sun also converts cholesterol found in your skin to vitamin D and its active forms. Unfortunately, you can't get that unless you go outside. The ultraviolet light (UV-B) that powers these conversions is blocked by window glass, and by sunscreen.[17]

Sunlight has gotten something of a bad rap because depletion of the atmosphere's ozone layer has resulted in a subsequent rise in incidence of melanoma, as well as basal cell and squamous cell carcinoma. This cannot be denied. However, sunlight can also help prevent a number of internal organ cancers and is a strong stimulus for a potent subset of T-regulator cells that reduce autoimmune phenomena, including type-1 diabetes and multiple sclerosis (which may explain why multiple sclerosis is so rare in southern climates). It may also be the basis of the selective migration of lighter-skinned people northward in prehistoric times, where the better protected darker skin does not admit enough sunlight for vitamin D conversion. Eskimos, the apparent exception, have diets especially rich in fish oils.[18]

In the Earth's temperate regions, the amount of UV-B available varies by a factor of 35 between July and December. In winter in Hungary, for example, it would be necessary to run around for more than two hours, one before and one just after noon, quite scantily clad, to get the requisite sunlight for adequate conversion. It is somewhat surprising that the entrepreneurial pharmaceutical firms have not made more of this fact when marketing the active forms of vitamin D.[19]

The proper dose of vitamin D is 400–800 international units daily.

Don't try to make up for lost time (or rays) by taking more than 1,500 units; an overdose actually can be fatal.

Additional daily nutritional needs include a number of metallic substances:

Magnesium (600 mg): The body's ability to absorb magnesium drops as it ages, and this critical component of hydroxyapatite is excreted even more if you drink alcohol or take diuretics. Magnesium is a necessary part of the body's cycle for activating vitamin D, and deficiencies affect the way estrogen, parathyroid hormone, and calcitonin function. Licorice, coriander, and dandelion contain magnesium, as do almonds, brown rice, green vegetables, and milk. Overdoses cause nausea or diarrhea.

Copper (3–10 mg): Copper competes with calcium for absorption, so supplements for one might necessitate a supplement for the other, taken at separate times.

Strontium (0.5–3 mg): Strontium migrates to boney sites and is thought to be important.

Zinc (20 mg): Zinc is critical for osteoblasts' and osteoclasts' basic chemistry in making and resorbing bone.

Other substances and other vitamins include:

Boron (3 mg): Important for the proper effects of estrogen, calcium and magnesium retention, and a large number of other reactions. Fruits, vegetables, and nuts contain all you'll probably need. Overdoses occur at 30 times the recommended amount.

Silicon (1–2 mg): Essential for all connective tissue, including bone. Silicon makes up most of the dirt vegetables are grown in, and it is abundant in the four B's—beer, beets, bell peppers, and brown rice—as well as green leafy vegetables.

Manganese (5–10 mg): Manganese is part of the boney matrix and thus necessary for bone health. Whole grains, spinach, and pineapple juice are particularly rich in manganese.

Vitamins: Vitamins important to bone health include B_6 (pyridoxine, 5–25 mg), B_9 (folic acid, 400 mcg), B_{12} (cyanocobalamine, 1000 mcg),

C (60 mg), and K (100–300 mcg). Bell peppers give you B_6, B_{12} and C; green leafy vegetables give you K and B_9, but the most reliable source of B_{12} are meat, dairy products, eggs, and vitamin pills.

These dietary suggestions are worth noting, but foods without these nutrients need not be eliminated! Eat what appeals to you, and check that you have these vitamins and minerals covered. All food has something of value to you, and let's face it: People have been around a lot longer than vitamin pills. However, most of us do not get the kind of workout you get hunting and gathering; we're living a lot longer now, and we're doing incredible things in those extra years.[20]

New Findings

Laboratory studies that support bone-building powers of new substances have begun to show up in the literature. Korean safflower (*Carthamus tinctorius* L.), for example, appears to raise a number of biochemical markers associated with bone synthesis.[21] Another study, this one of 60 rats bereft of sex organs and the hormones they produce, found that dried plums keep the trabeculae normal and prevent osteopenia for ninety days. Dried plum was found to augment an insulin-like growth factor (IGF-1), which we met before, while down-regulating a biochemically important factor (RANKL) that sustains osteoclasts. The same mechanism is believed to be at work in some of the medicines that treat osteopenia.[22]

These two substances, safflower oil and dried plum, both may enhance bone growth while slowing its destruction. It is important to note that these studies were

SUMMARY OF VITAMINS AND MINERALS WITH SUGGESTED DAILY INTAKE

Calcium 1,200–1500 mg
Vitamin D 400–800 IU
Sunlight 20 minutes at least
Vitamin B_6 (pyridoxine) 5–25 mg
Vitamin B_9 (folic acid) 400 mcg
Vitamin B_{12} (cyanocobalamine) 1,000 mcg
Vitamin C 60 mg
Vitamin K 100–300 mcg
Magnesium 600 mg
Zinc 20 mg
Manganese 5–10 mg
Copper 3–10 mg
Boron 3 mg
Silicon 1–2 mg
Strontium 0.5–3 mg

done only on rats, and that only the *markers* of bone deposition and reabsorption were observed. Before placing too much trust in these findings, it would be nice to see some bone density readings in human beings. Exactly how these substances figure into the mechanisms of growth and resorption needs elucidation, and the possible side effects of these and other nutritional supplements should be carefully evaluated in future studies.

A recent study that did measure bone density found that men taking a certain type of diuretic lost three times as much bone as other men, even though both groups had the same underlying condition, hypertension. In the sample of 3,300 men, whose bone density was measured over four and a half years, those taking Lasix and other "loop of Henle" diuretics lost 0.78 percent of their bone density, while nonusers lost only 0.33 percent. Occasional users of diuretics lost 0.58 percent.[23] Here one can see the virtue of drug trials.

Don'ts

Just as there are sins of omission, at times omitting things can be a virtue. But the "don'ts" without the "do's" are insufficient. There is a cartoon picturing two puzzled-looking cave men sitting on a rock. The caption reads "I don't understand it. The air is totally clean, our water is crystal clear, everything we eat is organic, but we still die at 28."

If you have kidney disease, ask your physician before taking supplements, especially calcium, magnesium, or silicon.

Salt uses up calcium when it is excreted; limit daily salt intake to 2,000 mg.[24]

Avoid smoking; more than two alcoholic drinks per day, one carbonated beverage (or none), one cup of coffee; and more than 5 to 6 ounces of protein a day. Protein metabolism requires calcium—the body loses 30–40 mg of calcium for each ounce of protein it digests.[25]

Counterintuitively, most vegetarians, getting adequate but relatively less protein, are actually less prone to osteoporosis than carnivores.

Another vegetarian-favoring fact is that animal fat reduces bone formation.

To summarize this chapter, we have constructed a list of the different factors that influence fractures and how much control we have over each. Items are assigned 0 if we have no control over them; 1 if we have some control, and 2 if we have full control under usual conditions. Items marked with an asterisk (*) are recognized as increasing risk by the National Osteoporosis Foundation, the American Association of Clinical Endocrinologists, and the North American Menopause Society.

HELPS	HURTS
High estrogen 1	History of a fracture 0*
Hormonal regularity 1	Low estrogen 1*
High testosterone 1	Scoliosis 1
Balanced parathyroid hormone 1	Digestive disorders 1
Balanced thyroid hormone 1	Anorexia nervosa 1
Adequate calcium 2	Depression 1
Adequate vitamin D 2	Glucocorticoids (anti-inflammatory) 1*
Adequate vitamins B 2	Chemotherapy 1
Adequate vitamin C 2	Antiseizure meds 1
Adequate exercise 2	Lithium (for bipolar disorder) 1
Good posture 2	Anticoagulants (antibloodclotting) 1
Sufficient, not excessive, protein 2	Loop diuretics (e.g., Lasix) 1
Adequate exposure to the sun 1	Poor vision 1*
Diclofenac (Voltaren, an NSAID) 1	Caucasian or Asian 0
Hydrochlorothiazide (diuretic) 1	Small stature 0**
Naproxen (Naprosyn, an NSAID) 1	History of falls 1*
African American background 0	Not bearing children 1
	Tobacco use 2*
	Alcohol use 2*

**We have yet to see a study that takes into account the fact that smaller people don't, on the average, fall as far or as hard.

Items with 0 are the ones that should motivate you; you have to make up for them. Those with a 1 encourage you to do what you can.

With number 2 the message is clear: Make the appropriate lifestyle changes.

Chapter 4

Medications for Osteoporosis

All right, you knew that it would have been better to go out for tennis when you were in seventh grade and train for track in high school, mind your minerals in your teens, and exercise big time after college. You're not a heavy drinker and you quit smoking, but now you *have* osteoporosis. What to do? Is it too late?

The dietary considerations outlined in chapter 3 apply to people who have osteopenia or osteoporosis as well as those who just want to avoid it. Vitamin D is for everyone. Lifestyle choices play a hefty part too. But let's turn to medications, which are reserved for the people that actually have low or rapidly falling bone mineral density. The medicines presented here are only for the 200-million-plus people who have that problem. Since you'll have to consult a physician, and his or her judgment is the one you listen to (or you must get another doctor), we focus on the medicines themselves, not when and whether you should take them.

Fosamax (Alendronate)

Fosamax was the first modern drug to treat osteoporosis that really took hold of the American medical community. At this writing in 2009 it is still the most frequently prescribed, though it was introduced many years ago and a number of other medications have been developed since. It is a bisphosphonate, a class of drugs that inhibit the osteoclasts, the cells that reabsorb calcium from bones. In osteopenia and osteoporosis, osteoclasts destroy bone faster than osteocytes lay it down. Fosamax slows down the destruction. That can tip the balance, and in a study of 3,658 women, Fosamax reduced the incidence of hip, vertebral, and wrist fractures by 53 percent, 45 percent, and 31 percent respectively.[1]

A randomized placebo-controlled Canadian study shows that alendronate is as effective in men as it is in women, regardless of the men's male (or female) hormone levels, or the magnitude of the patients' bone resorption. In either gender, patients' BMDs usually gain 6 percent in the first year of use and 2 percent each year thereafter. Ninety-five percent of the patients who have participated in clinical trials of this drug show a significant increase in BMD. The risk of any kind of fracture goes down about 50 percent. The usual dose is 5 mg daily for osteopenia, 10 mg per day for osteoporosis.[2]

The most common side effects are gastrointestinal. Patients are advised to stay clear of food for at least an hour after taking the medication. Acid reflux, nausea, and irregular bowels, along with muscular, abdominal, and bone pain, are the main things to worry about, and they are not uncommon. Other side effects, such as osteonecrosis (disintegration of the jawbone, auditory canal, or other bones) and slower healing of fractures that do occur have been discussed in the media over the past few years, but are estimated to be quite unusual, related to dental surgery, cancerous conditions, and the duration of treatment. In addition, there is evidence that bisphosphonates stay in the body for long periods of time, possibly throughout life, and can cross the placenta.[3]

This does not sound so bad. Few osteoporotic patients are of childbearing age, and don't you want the good effects to stay around and help you for a long time? Unfortunately the adverse effects are strong enough, or patients' resolve is weak enough, that compliance is a major issue. One recent study found that less than 35 percent of the people given prescriptions for this medication actually stay on it long enough to make it "therapeutically relevant."[4]

Actonel (Risedronate)

A second bisphosphonate, Actonel, has many of the same negative side effects as Fosamax, but it is a coated capsule. This lowers the chance of esophageal irritation.[5]

Boniva (Ibandronate)

More recently, and possibly because of the low compliance seen with the other bisphosphonates, Boniva, a once-a-month oral or injectible drug, has been introduced.

Ibandronate works the same way the other two bisphosphonates do, slowing down the resorption of bone by osteoclasts, but is so powerful that patients are strongly advised not to take it unless they are also taking calcium and vitamin D to supply the building blocks for healthy bone, have no kidney problems that would disturb their bodies' relatively constant levels of serum calcium, and can remain vertical for at least an hour after taking the medicine to minimize gastrointestinal side effects. Major adverse effects include abdominal pain, hypertension, joint pain, nausea, upset stomach, and diarrhea.

Reclast (Zoledronic Acid)

Recently things have gotten even simpler. Reclast, perhaps the ultimate bisphosphonate, is given as an annual intravenous infusion. Only 5 mg have proven 50 percent more effective than Actonel in treating people with osteoporosis acquired through exposure to steroids, and over four times more effective in building bone mass as a preventive measure.[5] Atrial fibrillation is a major adverse effect.

Regardless of which bisphosphonate one chooses, it is always wise to use calcium and vitamin D supplements as well. These nutritional supplements are used by controls and intervention patients in most of the studies that support the efficacy of these medications.[6]

Denosumab

As of 2009, denosumab is not yet on the market. Denosumab is an antibody that prevents the activator molecule RANKL from stimulating cells to evolve into osteoclasts, therefore reducing bone resorption. Side effects reported were few, and the gastric upset that is commonly associated with oral bisphosphonate use was substantially reduced. Increase in bone mass was greater with denosumab than with alendronate in a study of 412 patients, and bone synthesis was in full swing after only three days. Early trials have begun to find separate cortical and trabecular effects, and also indicate that the drug slows the development of rheumatoid arthritis.[7] A recent radiological study using densitometry and examination of bone structure suggests that denosumab actually improves bone quality.[8]

Estrogen, Progesterone, and Selective Estrogen Receptor Modulators (SERMs)

Hormone replacement therapy after menopause (HRT), seemed to be in the headlines almost every day for a while. Women commonly used it to tame the changes that come with menopause. Many conflicting studies associate HRT with an increased risk of uterine and breast cancer, heart disease, and thrombosis, but also with an improvement in bone mineral density. Birth control medications, premenopausal (and pharmaceutically quite different) forms of HRT, keep their users' bones quite youthful much of the time. A popular compromise solution is for menopausal women to take half the usual HRT dose, either orally or transcutaneously through a skin patch. The patch, enables the body to acquire the estrogen and/or progesterone without the hormones passing through the liver. Progesterone alone increased the bone mineral density of first-year users up to 10 percent with approximately 4 percent improvements each year thereafter.

Progesterone medications are frequently combined with estrogens such as estriol, estradiol, and estrone. Of these, 17 alpha-estriol appears to be the least toxic, actually reducing the progress of breast cancer, and the one of all of the estrogens that has a very low likelihood of re-initiating monthly menstruation.

Evista (Raloxifene)

This is an interesting medication that some, but not all, of the body's cells see and treat just as they do estrogen. Bone cells respond as they would to estrogen, reducing reabsorption of calcium, but other tissues are actually blocked by this drug from responding to any estrogen that the body happens to have around. It does not have estrogen's effect on the heart, and actually decreases the risk of breast cancer. The same risk of blood clots associated with estrogen use does seem to come with Evista.

Similar medications, such as lasofoxifene, bazedoxifene, and arzoxifene, were in clinical trials in 2009. Bazedoxifene was approved by the FDA in 2007 and will probably be available by early 2010 under the tradename Viviant; it may be combined with conjugated estrogens. Aprela, the combination medication, is currently in mid-trial (a Phase III study). Lasofoxifene has been approved in Europe by the CHMP and has received committee approval from the FDA. Eli Lilly has stopped work on arzoxifene.

Miacalcin (Calcitonin)

Contrary to the once-popular song, the hip bone is connected to the bloodstream. We have already reviewed the perils of too-low concentration of calcium in the bloodstream which include massive muscle spasm and may affect the smooth muscle of the heart. The body is therefore totally justified in ruthlessly appropriating calcium from the bones, where more than 90 percent of the body's calcium resides, in order to keep the whole organism running and intact. Calcitonin, a hormone synthesized in the thyroid gland, regulates and reduces the body's tendency to reabsorb the bones' calcium.

Just as estrogen and progesterone levels dwindle later in life, calcitonin levels fall as well. Salmon calcitonin is frequently used to supplement our natural supply, since it is much more potent than our own. Fish, of course, even the valiant salmon, have a different relationship with gravity, and have bones that are mainly muscle-strain-bearing, rather than weight-bearing. This may account for the fabulous power of the salmon calcitonin. More than 60 percent of the users of Miacalcin can expect improvement, often up to a 4 percent increase of bone mineral density, and 40 percent reduction in risk of fracture. It may be taken as a nasal spray, wherein lies its main but uncommon side effect, nasal irritation.

Being a biological product, Miacalcin is probably the drug of choice if gastric or other side effects prohibit the bisphosphonates, and cancer or other risks forbid hormone replacement therapy.

Forteo (Teriparatide)

Synthetic parathyroid hormone, teriparatide appears to increase bone mineral density and reduce vertebral and nonvertebral fractures without a substantial risk of raising calcium in the bloodstream to dangerous levels. It does this by tipping the balance in favor of bone build-up and slightly against bone breakdown. Both lower and higher doses of parathyroid hormone appear to favor build-up, but high doses (40 mg) were actually found to promote resorption at the forearm.[9] A Harvard study of 1,637 patients found that once-a-day injections of 40 mg were only slightly more effective than 20 mg, but had a greater likelihood of causing nausea and headache, the other chief side effects.[10]

Besides vitamin D, parathyroid hormone is the only other known naturally occurring substance that in and of itself will build bone.[11]

Horse before Cart

Dr. George Kessler points out that three quarters of the people taking medicines for osteoporosis do not take calcium and vitamin D daily.[12] He likens this to a contractor who has the electrician, the plumber, the roofers, the carpenters, and all the workmen assembled at a job site, but then does not deliver the electrical wires, the pipes, the shingles, or the lumber.

There are undeniable and also unpredictable side effects to all these medications. Although they are effective for prevention as well as remediation of low bone mineral density, those people with less than 2.5 standard deviation loss of bone might be wise to avoid them, in favor of a regimen that includes vitamin D, calcium, and exercise for a year or two, and then repeat a DEXA scan before embarking on any of the more rigorous and risky medical treatments. If there is substantial improvement, medication may not be necessary.

Chapter 5

Exercise

E xercise has been shown to improve the production of bone without affecting the rate of reabsorption. Once again an ounce of prevention is worth more than its weight in gold. There are steps you can take at any age, but earlier is better. Age five is not too soon. The late teens, even the postgraduate years, are not too late. But more to the point: Exercise is good at any age, and it's always better than inactivity.

From here onward, exercise is what this book is about. Almost any exercise is better than none, but some activities are especially beneficial. There are questions in the literature about weight-bearing exercises versus those that involve dynamic tension. Some types of exercise pose an agonizing dilemma: Those that help arthritis may worsen osteoporosis, and vice versa. Nevertheless, we know it is good to stretch and move.

Exercise has many benefits: It improves cardiac status, reduces the risk of breast cancer, lowers cholesterol, normalizes blood sugar, promotes weight loss, eases depression, builds muscle, and enhances balance, endurance, and pulmonary function. Some rigorous exercise is necessary for the creation and retention of strong bones.

Unlike drugs and many nutritional supplements, the side effects of exercise are all desirable. For example, in July 2008 the journal *Nature* contained an article describing PGC1 alpha, a cellular molecule that is generated through exercise. It is a powerful anti-inflammatory, reducing the incidence of a number of cancers, type-II diabetes, autoimmune illnesses, and Alzheimer's disease.[1] But there is no need to wait until results come back from the National Institutes of Health. A biologist once remarked that whatever an animal is doing now, one thing is sure: in a little while it will be doing something else. We are built for movement and change. All of our organs need activity to thrive. But we have the opportunity to pick exercises carefully. Many studies have found that moderate resistance activities conducted three times weekly for 6 to 24 months yield modest gains in bone mineral density; 0.006 gm/cm^2 in the spine, but not even that much in the hip. Fifteen studies of walking 90 to 280 minutes 3 to 5 times per week came to the same conclusion: slightly enhanced vertebral bone density without consistent improvement at the hip.[2]

One has to examine the results of the exercise studies carefully. Without much information about bone quality, many studies may be misleading. It is possible that some exercises cause bones to remodel and strengthen their structure without changing their density. After all, we know that during the first three years of life, when we are learning to walk, the thigh bone normally angles itself inward more than 60 degrees at the hip, proving that the angular stress of walking is a powerful force in bone formation (see page 58).[3]

Muscle Strength

Muscular strength is important both for building bones and for resisting falls, particularly in older people. Fifty healthy postmenopausal women had two supervised 60–70 minute exercise sessions and two 25-minute unsupervised sessions per week for a little over two years. Both they and a control group were given calcium and vitamin D; none of the women were taking medication. Both groups were tested at the beginning and end of the study for bone mineral density, cholesterol, and general level of fitness. BMD did not change significantly in the exercise group, but decreased in the control group in spite of the calcium and vitamin D supplements. In every measurement of bone density, the exercisers outstripped the declining controls, sometimes by as much as 7 percent in that short period of time. The exercise group had modestly lower blood cholesterol and reported less pain.[4] Strength was another part of the story: Trunk flexors and extensors gained more than 35 percent in the exercise group. Strength measures were essentially flat in the nonexercising controls. Cholesterol and triglyceride levels were 9.1 percent and 37.4 percent in the right direction in the exercise group, and the opposite for both in the controls.[5]

A specific form of exercise, spinal extensions or back bends, appears to be more advantageous and less dangerous than, for example, spinal flexion exercises—forward bends—for people with osteoporosis. A number of studies conducted by Meersheed Sinaki and her group at the Mayo Clinic suggest that spinal extension exercises are safer than flexion exercises, the latter increasing the incidence of vertebral fractures.[6] The forward, hump-like curve that often develops as we age is exaggerated by bending forward, increasing the pressure and therefore the risk of vertebral fracture. Flexion exercises such as sit-ups shorten the radius of spinal curvature, and over time will strengthen the muscles that produce it. As this process continues, more and more weight gets concentrated at the front of the vertebral bodies, and the stronger the muscles get, the greater the forces they generate on an ever-reducing area of bone.[7] If 100 pounds of pressure are concentrated on one square inch of bone, that's 100 pounds per square inch. But if the bones are acutely tipped forward, that same 100 pounds on one tenth of an inch will produce 1,000 pounds of pressure per square inch on that small fraction of the bone. And, of course, as you strengthen the muscles, the forces themselves will rise too.

But algebra, geometry, and physics are not the whole story. Leonardo da Vinci reasoned long ago that because a bone's strength is related to its cross-sectional area (πr^2), and an animal's weight is related to its volume ($4/3 \, \pi \, r^3$), and since healthy bone has a fairly constant density and strength, and we are composed chiefly of water, the ratio of any healthy animal's bone length to thickness should be a specific, constant value. But in every case ever examined, da Vinci was wrong. He treated body structure as an engineer or architect might, as a static edifice, like a column or buttress. But in living things, gravity is not the only, nor even the most prominent influence on body structure. Muscular movement is far more powerful.[8]

We overcome gravity in almost everything we do, from lifting our little fingers to pole vaulting. Further, our muscles often oppose one another, greatly increasing the stimulating strain on the bones. This happens especially in more highly skilled, even delicate, measured movements. Just think of holding a pencil, washing your feet, doing a pantomime, clapping. Using health club devices, wrestling, and swimming under water each presents its own type of resistance. In each activity, movement is only possible because our muscles are stronger than whatever forces oppose them.

Many people still believe that weight-bearing is the best, perhaps only, type of exercise for building bones, but that is patently false. One need only consider the fine glistening bones of non-weight-bearing fish to recognize that the truth is otherwise. One need go no farther than his or her own arm, wrist, and fingers to find examples of non-weight-bearing bones that may become osteoporotic, but usually don't in spite of the absence of weight-bearing in all but yogis and acrobats. There is a physiological principle that has been around for more than one hundred years which explains all this. Wolff's law, the basis of bone-shaping, states that the architectural strength of a bone develops along the lines of force to which that bone is subjected. This makes physiological sense, because it means that a bone will develop reinforcement to counter exactly the stresses and strains that it undergoes. This explains why our arms are doing so well and why yoga can help us manage osteoporosis. Even though the arms are not weight bearing, these bones are constantly

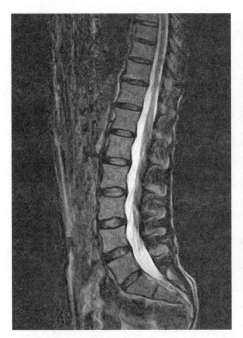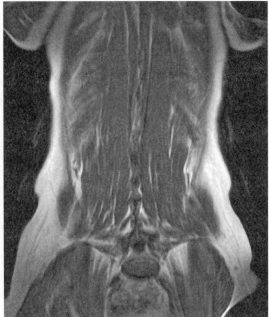

Figure 15. *Stress stimulates bones to strengthen. Yoga appears to mend the damage and asymmetries from the buffets endemic to life. Witness the beautiful spine of this 16-year yoga practitioner and teacher.*

exposed to the pull of muscles in daily life activities such as carrying groceries or playing tennis.

Wolff's law may also have bearing on the question running though a good deal of current research: Is bone quality, the combination of BMD and the structural elements of bone, affected by exercise in a meaningful way?

When a child is born, the heads of his or her thigh bones are perfectly straight, much like the equivalent bones in the upper arm. But after walking becomes a habitual and customary means of locomotion, the femur begins to develop an angle, straightened only from the greater trochanter, where muscles intervene to impose another force that directly counters and significantly exceeds gravity. In the unfortunate children that congenitally cannot walk, this characteristic angle of the head of the thigh

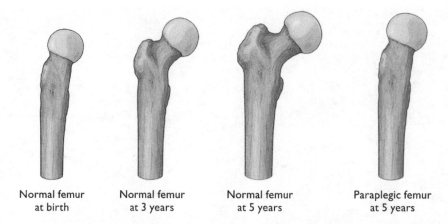

| Normal femur | Normal femur | Normal femur | Paraplegic femur |
| at birth | at 3 years | at 5 years | at 5 years |

THE CHANGING SHAPE OF THE FEMUR IN RESPONSE TO WEIGHT-BEARING

Figure 16. *The flying-buttress-like development of the hip bone is a response to the abductors holding the body up while the opposite leg swings forward in normal gait, cantilevering the body as it does so. With bone buildup between the joint and the lever arm, at the greater trochanter, the shaft itself gradually takes on a greater angle. In paraplegia these forces are never brought to bear, and the femur stays in its original linear form.*

bone never forms, and the inutile femur remains straight as an arrow throughout life.

Bone reinforces itself along the lines of stress generated by walking. The shaft of the femur actually migrates, lining up along lines of stress, until it opposes gravitational force enough to minimize further migration. Then, as though following a script, the migration stops. Yes, our activity has a powerful effect on bone formation. Now we must focus on that fascinating principle.

Chapter 6

A Wollf in Yoga Clothing

This story begins as an engineer wanders into a museum of natural history in the city of Cologne, Germany, where he is commissioned to build a crane. He notices that the areas of reinforcement in the bones of a vulture's wing have exactly the same form and pattern as the head of the crane he is designing.

The small article he publishes about this remarkable similarity is read by Julius Wollf, a surgeon and anatomist, who looks into the matter. He studies many different bones; the pattern of reinforcement seems to be a widespread phenomenon. A few years later, in 1892, he writes a book on the subject. He puts forward a theory to explain the wonderful job nature does throughout the phylum Chordata, which includes all creatures with bones and spinal cords: Bones strengthen just where they need it the most.[1]

He formulates a principle that encapsulates the order he has found in nature. Wollf's law states that the architectonic of a bone, its underlying structural system of support, follows the lines of force to which that bone is subjected.

If loading on a particular bone increases, the bone will remodel itself over time to become stronger and resist that sort of loading. The converse is true as well: If the loading on a bone decreases, the bone will adapt and become lighter and weaker. Numerous studies have found that pressure on the bones is a potent force responsible for bone shape and strength.[2]

Forces That Strengthen Bone

What produces those pressures? How do they come about; how do they come to bear on the fate of our bones? Let's begin with a couple of examples.

- Muscular stimulus. Bones in the racket-holding arms of tennis players become much stronger than the bones in the opposite arm, since those bones are routinely under stress.
- Gravity. Astronauts who spend a long time in space will often return to Earth with weaker bones, since their muscles have had no opposition—gravity hasn't been exerting any load. Their bodies have reabsorbed much of the mineral that was in their bones.

Gravity is not the only force, nor the strongest force, acting upon bones. Although gravity is certainly a power to be reckoned with and an important element in maintaining bone strength and design, two other forces must, by their very nature, be stronger: mechanical leverage and dynamic tension.

Mechanical leverage is produced by our anatomy. Every 45-pound child knows that if Dad sits close enough to the cross-bar of the teeter-totter, he or she can lift 180 pounds. Many muscles, such as the quadriceps, insert close to the joint they cross, making for considerable leverage. For example, the supraspinatus, located at the edge of the shoulder, attaches to the very tip of the humerus, yielding pressures that are fifty times greater than any weight lifted by the straight arm. This mechanical advantage can multiply gravity's force many times over.

Dynamic tension occurs when one muscle or muscle group opposes

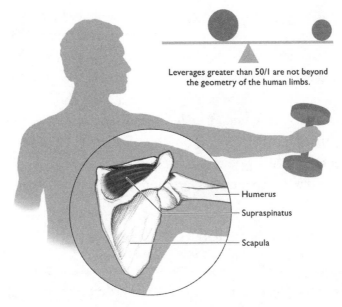

Leverages greater than 50/1 are not beyond
the geometry of the human limbs.

Humerus

Supraspinatus

Scapula

THE LEVERAGE OF THE SUPRASPINATUS MUSCLE

Figure 17. *This leverage greatly amplifies the force to which the bone is exposed.*

the action of another, and not coincidentally this happens when practicing most yoga poses. The force created is greater than gravity. Since there are two groups of muscles applying opposite pressure, the forces on the bones are doubled. Astronauts could minimize muscle loss, and therefore osteoporosis, by doing yoga in space.

Muscular activity stimulates bones to strengthen themselves much more vigorously than weight-bearing alone, and in so doing can protect the bones from inordinate thinning. This effect seems to operate even in conditions of calcium deficiency.[3] Contemporary science has traced and verified the phenomenom just about every step of the way; a convincing number of biochemical markers of the bone-building process have been measured before and after different activities that involve dynamic tension. One biochemical marker, 3H-uridine, is relatively easy to measure. Its level increased six times over levels seen in resting tissue after pressure was applied to bones both in the laboratory and in live animals.[4] The duration of the pressure is an important factor as well. In another study it took only eight seconds of dynamic loading to initiate physiologic processes that prevent weakening of bone.[5] In yoga, we hold poses for longer than eight seconds.

That is one of the reasons yoga is such a good choice for preventing bone density problems, and for reducing existing ones: Yoga positions are held for periods of time; there is not the constant shifting that you see in tennis, biking, and many other sports. Through yoga practice, the bone has the stimulus duration required to promote the processes of strengthening.

Mechanoreception, Wherein Lies the Magic

We have seen how osteoblasts come to surround themselves with the protein they secrete, and before long have become almost totally isolated

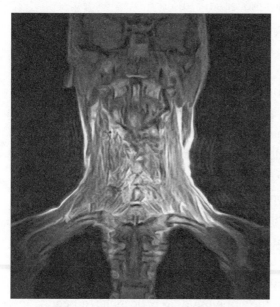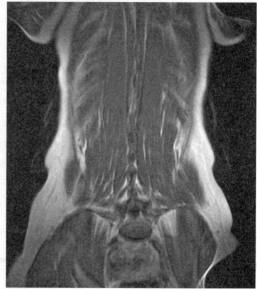

Figure 18. *Frontal MRI views of cervical (left) and lumbar (right) spinal musculature. Cervical and cranial muscles insert largely on the scapulae, clavicles, and sternum. Using the arms to lift or support weight gives stimulating compression to the cervical vertebrae. The same applies to the muscles that interconnect the bodies and transverse processes of the lumbar vertebrae.*

from other similar cells. At this point they change from oval osteoblasts to star-shaped osteocytes. One of their new functions is to maintain the collagen-plus-calcium that makes up the bone. Another is to secrete the new protein matrix on which new bone forms. The key to this entire process is mechanoreceptors: tiny parts of the cell wall that respond to movement by altering the cell's function. Tiny hairs that protrude from receptor cells in the ears, responsible for turning vibrations of air into the sounds we hear, are an example. All the nerve cells that let us know when something touches us and convey sensations of movement are in this category. Mechanoreceptors react to some physical impingement, something that jostles or juts against the membrane, the sound or the touch, by sending an impulse to the brain. At the ear, we do not "feel" the vibration, we hear it. On the skin, we are not aware of how deep an impression a commuter handle makes when we grasp it; we feel the cold metal and its shape, that's all. The actual moving of cell membranes goes on at the microscopic level. Mechanoreceptors have probably been part of cells for a very long time. They appear in primitive bacteria and fungi, suggesting that they occurred in a common ancestor; the division of these two fundamental categories of life happened some 3.5 billion years ago.

Osteocytes are a third example of mechanoreceptors. We don't generally know that our bones are being bent or twisted, yet many studies document that this is exactly what happens. While lifting, carrying, steering, stooping, the bones arch and torque under every strain. When the osteocytes' outer membranes are stretched or squeezed, as they are by any bending or twisting of the bone itself, they quickly react by synthesizing more of the protein spicules that make up the matrix of new bone.

Osteocytes extend long tentacles, greatly increasing their surface area and the regions in which they are sensitive to positional change.[6] A change in the shape, however slight, of a cell's outer surface alters its inner metabolism and function. Most commonly, tiny electric charges generated by the membrane's movement supply energy sufficient to change messenger molecules at the cell membrane's interior. These molecules then make their way to the nucleus. There they fit into the nuclear membrane in a

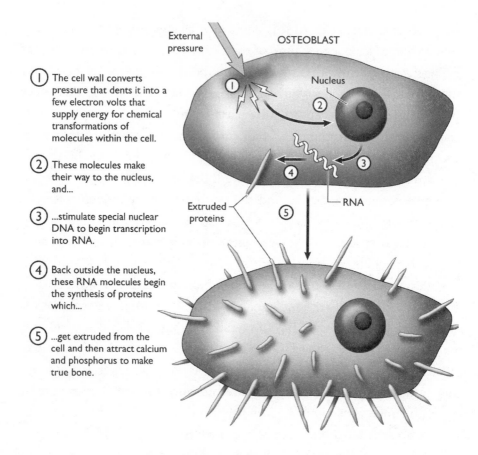

The cell wall converts pressure that dents it into a few electron volts that supply energy for chemical transformations of molecules within the cell.

These molecules make their way to the nucleus, and...

...stimulate special nuclear DNA to begin transcription into RNA.

Back outside the nucleus, these RNA molecules begin the synthesis of proteins which...

...get extruded from the cell and then attract calcium and phosphorus to make true bone.

AN OSTEOBLAST'S RESPONSE TO EXERCISE

Figure 19. *Deformation of the cell wall triggers electron discharges that initiate chemical reactions, forming specific molecules at the cell wall's inner surface. These molecular signals diffuse throughout the cell, reaching to the cell's nucleus. The nucleus responds by transcribing a new batch of DNA into RNA, which in turn makes new proteins. These are then extruded from the cell into the boney matrix, attracting minerals that strengthen the bone exactly where the strain originally occurred, reducing further deformation.*
After Junqueira and Carniero, p. 156, with permission of the publisher.

way that influences the nuclear processes themselves. Almost like a neurotransmitter, these tiny messengers from the cell's outer border affect its very core; they change the DNA, RNA, and the proteins made by the cell thereafter, transforming what the cell can send out into the body. In the case of osteocytes, the process leads to synthesis of more bone-making protein that is then extruded by the cell into the boney matrix surrounding it. The matrix attracts calcium and other minerals that strengthen the bone, and subsequently damp down the movement of the osteocytes' membranes. This in turn stiffens the bone against bending, which cuts the stimulation for new bone to form. The entire process is the biochemical basis for Wolff's law.[7]

What pressure does for the osteocytes, it seems to do for cartilage as well. Perhaps this is not startling since the cells that create bone and those that create cartilage both develop from mesenchymal stem cells. Surprising or not, understanding the process does form a fuller picture of yoga's advantages: You can strengthen bone by opposing one muscle to another, and renew cartilage by applying no-impact stress and increasing range of motion. In this way, yoga may reduce osteoporosis, and osteoarthritis as well.

There is another noteworthy aspect of mechanoreception that Wolff anticipated: Osteocytes respond locally to motion exactly along the axis where the bone is bending, making it resistant to that very bending. As the process continues and the bone strengthens itself against that stress, there is less bending, and the buildup is moderated. This feedback loop keeps bones from outgrowing their usefulness: They are stimulated to thicken at a given point to the extent that is necessary to minimize bending, and no further. The process modulates the creation and destruction cycle of osteocytes and osteoclasts, allowing only enough bending to stimulate bone-building equal to the destruction wrought by osteoclasts.

The same consideration also explains why eccentric pulls, stretches against some resistance (like those that occur so commonly in yoga), are particularly useful. The bone mineral density relates to all-around thickness of the bone. Eccentric, unusual pulls stimulate bone in many more places, thickening and strengthening it overall, protecting it from many points of impact or strain. Opposing the bone's long axis with unusual stresses, as all of yoga's bends and extensions do, is bound to stimulate new bone production. For these reasons it is likely to be particularly effec-

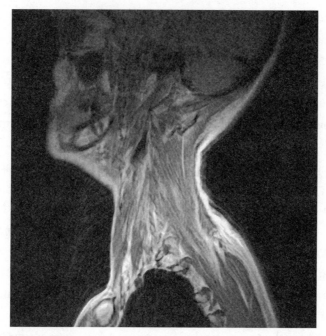

Figure 20. *The muscles of the lateral neck and head can stimulate the cervical vertebrae in almost every conceivable direction.*

tive against the compression fractures that commonly damage vertebrae, including six of the seven cervical vertebrae.

Calling on Wolff for Prevention and Treatment of Osteoporosis

Almost all experts agree that prevention of osteoporosis is more effective than treatment. Any diligent prevention regimen takes into account the arc that, with minor variation, charts out the natural history of thickening and subsequent weakening of every person's bones (see the graph of BMD vs. age on page 19). Beginning a yoga practice early in life—twenties, teens, even younger!—will help the bones strengthen at a time when conditions are maximal. Applying the pressures inherent in yoga will raise peak bone mass, maxing it out at a higher level. Add the benefits of cartilaginous and ligamentous irrigation that stretching and compression provide, and the greater range of motion that stretching obviously brings, there is a fairly compelling picture for yoga as preventive practice. (For more information on yoga as prevention and treatment for joint disease, see our book *Yoga for Arthritis*.)

We have been studying yoga's effect on bones for years. In our latest study we solicited men and women with osteopenia or osteoporosis through advertisements, and we also invited patients who had come to us for other reasons. Each patient gave blood and urine samples, so we could be sure that they had no metabolic conditions that would have an unpredictable effect on the results of the study. Each had a DEXA scan, unless they had completed one within the previous six months. We taught them ten yoga poses, designed for safety, that specifically strengthen the parts of the body most vulnerable to fracture: the lumbar and thoracic vertebrae, the hip, and the thigh. These are also the very places that the DEXA scan measures.

Some subjects came to our offices a number of times to learn the poses correctly; sometimes two or three sessions were enough. Others learned the poses with step-by-step instructions from our Web site, sciatica.org. We made contact with everybody every three to four months to find out how they were doing; to ask whether they were practicing the yoga, and if so, how much and how often; whether there had been any adverse effects; and, of course, to answer any questions. We modified the yoga poses for people who were stiff, or who had other medical conditions; some were able to upgrade their practices in time. We also began a monthly newsletter and bulletin board, both accessible from sciatica.org.

The study is still in progress. Even at this early point, the twelve people who have been doing yoga for two years to improve their bone mineral density have shown a statistically significant rise in their DEXA scores for both the vertebral column and the hip!

The study patients showed an increase in spine BMD equivalent to 0.563 units on the T-scale; their hip BMD increased 0.867 units. Control patients (those who were not practicing yoga) values were –0.12 and –0.07 for spine and hip respectively over the two-year study period. The patients

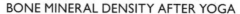

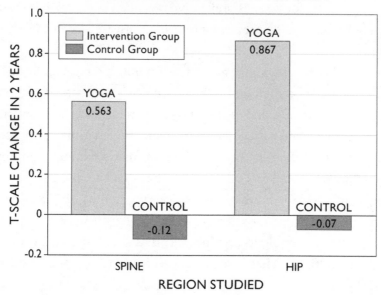

Figure 21. *In this two-year pilot study, those who practiced yoga improved BMD dramatically, while controls lost BMD. This difference is statistically significant.*

doing yoga gained enough bone in their spine to return most osteopenics' measurements to normal, and enough bone to restore a minimally osteoporotic hip nearer to the bone density of a healthy 25- to 30-year-old.

There were only seven patients in the control group, so we compared the boney gains of the twelve patients practicing yoga to the null hypothesis, the proposition that yoga did *not* improve bone mineral density. This is an overly stringent condition, going further than we need to go. These early findings are encouraging, to say the least. To learn more about the study, including our efforts to continue and expand it, see www .sciatica.org and click on the osteoporosis section in the left-hand column.

Chapter 7

Yoga Stands Apart

Almost any form of exercise appears to stimulate osteocytes somewhat. Provided you eat properly, are getting enough vitamin D and calcium, don't smoke, avoid chronic use of steroids, and stay clear of the other Don'ts listed in chapter 3, you can run, jog, pump iron, spike a volleyball, or ride horses. What's wrong with Jazzercize, kick boxing, and tennis? Has someone anointed yoga with a special oil?

Whatever you do has to be active. Acupuncture might be helpful in regulating hormones, but what you need to prevent the thinning of your bones cannot be done *to* you nor *for* you. This is something that *you* must do. All therapies can be broken up into three categories—passive, interactive, and active—a neat tripartite division that is relevant here.

Passive therapies are things that are done *to* you. There is generally an expert, often with a degree to show for his or her study. He or she does the therapeutic things that constitute massage or chiropractic treatment or prescribes the medicine or does the surgery that you receive. Acupuncture, and all the hormone therapies and other medicines

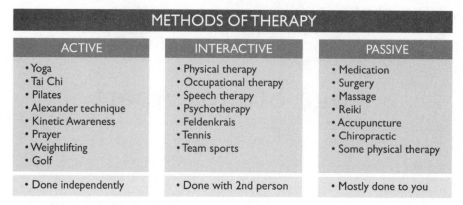

Figure 22. *Three categories of therapy, with a small number of representative disciplines in each one to illustrate their similarities and differences.*

reviewed earlier fit in here. When it comes to osteoporosis and the physical activity its treatment requires one should look further.

Interactive therapies take two, and one of the people involved generally has the lion's share of the expertise. But give-and-take is intrinsic to all of them, even if it is not always equal. In psychotherapy, for example, both parties are spectacularly inactive. If your view of interaction extends to all mammals, then horseback riding is an interactive therapy too, but it's clear who's doing most of the work. In group sports such as tennis or football, the interactive group may be quite demanding and active, but the nature of the interaction is unsuitable for people at risk of fracture and inefficient when certain bones or areas need special attention.

Active therapies are the ones you do yourself. You may have to learn them from someone, but after that you can practice on your own. Each can be done successfully alone. When the activity is done in a group such as golf, or in a class setting, as is often the case with yoga, one gets some instruction, but not much interaction. Essentially, it's parallel play.

In work with osteoporosis, the active therapies are the ones that make the most sense. These are the ones that are the most helpful and present the smallest risk. Let us take a look at some of them.

Tai chi has a fair range of movements and will improve balance.[1] It is moderately good at retaining but not at increasing strength. The pressures on bones, the angles and leverage in its fluid movements oppose no force much greater than gravity.

Originally developed for athletes, acrobats, and dancers, *Pilates* is a broad term now used to describe a range of activities focusing on everything from mind-body awareness to superhuman fitness. The aim of Pilates is to create stability and flexibility in movement, eliminate muscular and structural imbalances, and strengthen the core muscles of the body. Traditional Pilates involves a sequence of exercises with or without equipment, while nontraditional or intuitive Pilates is tailored to individual needs. Many Pilates exercises are derived from yoga poses. While there is no particular spiritual focus in Pilates, there is a strong emphasis on concentration and mindfulness.

Alexander technique focuses on posture, which is a definite component in osteoporosis and osteoporotic fractures and a potent preventative measure when it comes to falls. It has been shown to relieve pain quite effectively, and was heralded as the first holistic therapy. Nobelist Sir Charles Sherrington wrote: "Mr. Alexander has done a service to the subject by insistently treating each act as involving the whole integrated individual, the whole psychophysical man. To take a step is an affair not of this or that limb solely but of the total neuromuscular activity of the moment—not least of the head and neck."

In our experience the Alexander technique has been outstanding in relieving pain and improving gait and posture. But it is not particularly active. It makes little attempt at strengthening, or putting special pressure on bones.

Kinetic Awareness is another combination of physical and mental activity. The technique involves using the body's weight resting on rubber balls to create a suspended stretch and massage on localized areas of the body. No great forces are generated, but it has helped a number of our patients with spasm and pain. Its benefit in osteoporosis consists of helping to relieve the common types of musculoskeletal pain that often preclude exercise. Mobility improves, and thus there is a greater likelihood that an exercise program can succeed. In addition, Kinetic Awareness on the spine can help reduce kyphosis, or hunched posture, a major risk factor for vertebral fracture. Stretching of any kind will increase a person's range of motion, which means that more stimulus to the bones will occur during daily activities and exercise. However, Kinetic Awareness alone can hardly be expected to reverse osteoporosis.

Weight lifting surely does produce the forces. Weights are easy to obtain and use at home. No question about building strength either. The disadvantages are that lifting weights does not improve range of motion, do much for balance, or involve much stretching, through which cartilage thrives. Also, weight lifting can give rise to a number of orthopedic and disc-related injuries, from low back pain to shoulder dislocation. These are not only painful, but also can disable the practitioner from continuing.

Golf is a wonderful way to get the 20 minutes of sunlight required to convert vitamin D to its active form. It so enthralls millions of people that they go to driving ranges to practice hitting the long ball—a half hour that can be far more active than playing the game itself. Those twists must be pure manna for the osteocytes of the pelvis and spine and good for intervertebral cartilage as well. While walking 18 holes cannot be considered inactive, when it comes to improving your range of motion, your balance, and your strength, golf is under par.

Every one of these activities is preferable to inactivity, and with persistence and imagination, each can be adapted to give an individual what he or she needs. It's hard to picture Tiger Woods with osteoporosis, even at age 90. There's no question that each of these is good. Still, after a short inspection of yoga, many conclude it is the logical best choice to prevent and treat osteoporosis.

Although yoga can be slow, requiring months or even years to achieve major effects, the trip is pleasant and without side effects, overhead, or undertow. In osteoporosis treatment, most interventions take years to

WHAT IS GOOD ABOUT YOGA?

• Nontoxic

Since yoga is not a medication, you'd think this benefit is too obvious to state. But the impurities in the air we breathe, the water we drink, the carcinogenic potential of the very sunlight that bone-building requires, contrast with yoga, where it's hard to find a deleterious side effect. Injuries are few when taught by a competent teacher.

• Free

Unlike so many medical means of prevention and treatment, once learned, there's an option to take yoga classes at any time, but no necessity.

• Portable

As compared with weightlifting, golf, or just about any activity for which the person alone is not sufficient, in yoga the practitioner is the equipment.

• Ageless

One Swedish king is alleged to have played tennis at 93. But you can see centenarians doing yoga in every major city of the world every day.

• Time-tested

Like pebbles at the seashore, worn smooth by mutual friction in the ceaseless action of the waves, yoga poses have been perfected over long periods of time by a quiet, relentless, ancient process resembling evolution itself.

• Promotes independence

The yogic attitude expects little from others and a lot from oneself. There may be a teacher, but there need be no master, because the practitioner carries within him- or herself strength, calm, and balance. Yoga has no addictive component, no medicines, talismans, or indispensable people.

• Spiritual but not religious

Yoga's philosophy calls upon us to develop a humble sense of wonder, a reverence for life and a connection with the inner wisdom that may be the lifeblood of all religions. Yoga is theistic without any organized church or clerical hierarchy. So far as we know, it is consistent with every faith and has adherents within many religions. It is in favor of honesty, kindness, and self-understanding; it is against violence of any kind except self-defense.

THE DISADVANTAGES OF YOGA

• Least accessible to those who need it the most

The people who have never done yoga, who may enjoy rich diets and suffer poor ranges of motion, are the ones who would receive the greatest benefits from it, but are, naturally, the ones for whom it is least appealing. If this sounds like you, find an experienced, sympathetic, and resourceful teacher who knows where your abilities lie and is able to tap them to help you. Then give that teacher this book.

• Not a science

Until very recently articles about yoga had not been peer reviewed nor subject to cross-validation studies. The International Association of Yoga Therapists, the Annals of Internal Medicine, and the Journal of the American Medical Association, all peer-review journals, have begun to publish studies of the therapeutic benefits of yoga, some controlled, double blinded, and with state-of-the-art statistical analyses. But yoga itself is a practice, not a science. Its viewpoint is historically introspective, not empirical. To fully enter the mainstream, yet continue to provide the classical rewards, yoga therapy has the difficult but essential task of retaining its spiritual aspect while demonstrating measurable, replicable medical benefit.

• No lure of immediate gratification

Unlike most medications, all surgery, and most applications of acupuncture and chiropractic, yoga's benefits may take weeks, months, even years to appear. But this is not always the case. Beginners may feel elation after or even during their first experience.

show results. Research is just now beginning to show the benefits of yoga by the standard criteria of Western medicine. Because the practice is sometimes adopted with near-religious fervor, one may hear extravagant claims about yoga's powers, but like everything else, yoga is subject to evaluation. At present, we may at least rely on the legions of enthusiastic practitioners and teachers who attest to its effectiveness.[2]

The Link between Yoga and Skeletal Well-Being

Our nearly ubiquitous mechanoreceptors have been examined in their various locations throughout the body. In 1999 a group of Japanese investigators found that stimulating the mechanoreceptors in the cartilage of intervertebral discs with cyclic tensile stress increased the rate of DNA metabolism and enhanced the manufacture of new collagen.[2]

It is fascinating to note that ligaments, cartilage, intervertebral discs, and possibly a number of other softer tissues all develop by responding adaptively to pressures developed in movement. This idea goes some distance toward assuring those who have some doubt about the advisability of exercise; it is more evidence that we were made to move.

In another study, cyclic tensile stretch, a form of mechanical stress, greatly increased the rate of DNA synthesis in cartilage cells that make up the intervertebral discs. The increased rate of DNA synthesis led directly to an increase in collagen, a protein that makes up the cartilage of intervertebral discs.[3] There is reason, then, to believe that gentle but extreme movements of the kind so characteristic of yoga are helpful for the softer tissues of cartilage and ligaments as well as bone. Yoga, possibly unique in the active therapies, escapes being too meek to counter osteoporosis or so abrupt that it aggravates osteoarthritis (see figure 23).

On the mind-body border, yoga has been shown to reduce anxiety, relieve asthma, regularize brain wave rhythms and increase the thickness of the cortical layer in our brains, help lose weight, ease labor delivery, and stabilize marriages.[4]

Yoga promotes balance, increases range of motion and strength, improves manual learning skills, brings about relaxation, lowers blood pressure, counters spasticity, generates no impact, and stretches muscles against themselves, exerting many hundreds of pounds of pressure on the bones to which they are attached, but in a gradual, nontraumatic, and self-regulating way. One last thing: Yoga is interesting. There is no reason to distract yourself with a health club's 17 television channels; let the iPod fall silent. In learning what your body can do, becoming

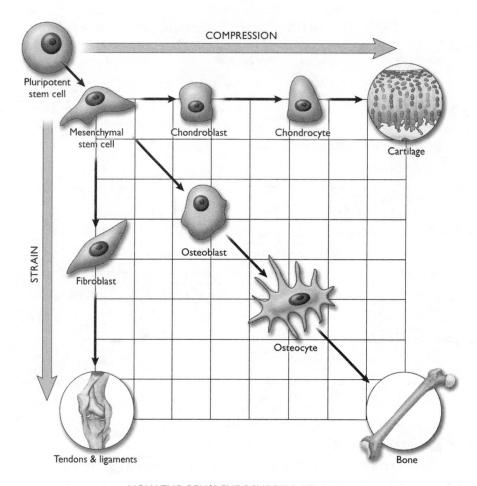

COMPRESSION

STRAIN

Pluripotent
stem cell

Mesenchymal
stem cell

Chondroblast

Chondrocyte

Cartilage

Osteoblast

Fibroblast

Osteocyte

Tendons & ligaments

Bone

HOW THE CELL'S EXPOSURE TO STRAIN AND
COMPRESSION DETERMINE ITS FUTURE

Figure 23. *Stem cells produce a variety of cells: from cells that make ligaments, to cells that secrete tendons, to those that produce cartilage, and the osteoblasts that are eventually embedded in bone. The uncommitted stem cells receive signals to develop one way or another according to the forces to which they are subjected, suggesting a corollary to Wolff's law. The forces are largely determined by their location. But all need activity to stay healthy. From T. Matsumoto, et al. "Cyclic mechanical stretch stress increases the growth rate and collagen synthesis of nucleus pulposus cells in vitro." Spine 24, no. 4: 315–319.*

acquainted with your muscles and joints, in quieting and eventually apprehending your mind, you may find yourself inherently fascinating. As Mr. Iyengar wrote many years ago, "Life's greatest adventure is getting to know yourself."[5]

We think yoga's the best; that's why we wrote the book. You may not know how you feel yet. What follows is the actual thing, the yoga. If the shoe fits, wear it boldly; it will take you where you want to go.

Chapter 8

Before You Start

Chronologically speaking, the rest of this book is written backward. We begin with poses for people that already have osteoporosis, and work our way through osteopenia back to people that have neither, and don't want them later in life. Because there are safety concerns that arise when learning yoga without a flesh-and-blood teacher, we start with the simplest and least precarious versions of all the poses, and build up from there. It would be an ironic catastrophe, but a catastrophe nonetheless, if some fastidious reader were to suffer the very fracture she or he is trying to avoid while doing what is intended to prevent it.

There are more than 15.5 million Americans practicing yoga as of this writing, and many of them have been doing it for years. Some may feel impatient when treated as a beginner. To these people we offer the following counsel: There is nothing as sophisticated as the fundamentals. Calmly read through these pages, and spend some time doing the more elementary versions of the poses, even if only to know them well enough to teach those who are less experienced or more vulnerable.

How the Poses Are Organized

Chapters 9, 10, and 11 each contain a set of yoga poses, all demonstrated at three levels of safety (except for the resting pose at the end). Each set comprises a complete array of stresses and stretches you'll need to combat osteoporosis and keep osteoarthritis at bay. Each promotes the three essential elements to preventing osteoporotic fractures, but each set has a different emphasis: the first group promotes bone solidity, the second aims more to build muscular strength, and the third focuses on balance. All three of these elements are critical for avoiding a fracture. If your deficit lies more in one of these areas than the others, spend more time practicing the poses that will address it. Choose that set and do it every day. You could also choose two groups and alternate. Another plan would be to do each group for two successive days, covering all three sets each week.

Chapter 9 includes poses that stimulate the bones in a variety of ways. It is critical that people with osteoporosis avoid kyphosis, a convex rounding of the spine. The "forward bend" poses in this group teach safe forward motion at the hips joints, which we call "folding," since bending of the spine is exactly what we're trying to avoid. Done correctly, folding stimulates the anterior vertebral bodies to produce stronger bone. The pressures that are brought to bear through the legs and hips also create a safe amount of gradually increasing stimulation that will strengthen and harden those bones against fracture. This first group, then, emphasizes bone solidity.

In chapter 10, the focus is on muscular strength—stronger thigh muscles in the standing poses, stronger arms and shoulders in the poses where they are recruited to work, and stronger abdominal and trunk muscles in such poses as Staff and Boat. Strength helps prevent falls and has the added benefit of allowing you to apply stronger, more stimulating forces to the bones.

Chapter 11 emphasizes balance, a critical attribute to develop in order to avoid falls. These poses require, and thereby build, agility and a sense of equilibrium.

Inside the Chapters

In all chapters, each pose is offered in three variations. The first variation is for those who already have a diagnosis of osteoporosis. The pressure on the bones will be mild yet effective, and these variations will safely prepare you to do the more difficult variations that follow. Pay special attention to the details of the instructions; it matters *how* you do the poses, not just which poses you do.

The second variation is intended for people with osteopenia. There is greater stress on the bones, but not so much as to approach anything unsafe for that condition.

The third variation is for people who do not have osteoporosis or osteopenia and would like to do what they can to avoid them. These are often the classical version of a yoga pose, or close to it.

Begin an orderly progression from the least challenging group that is appropriate for you. If the pilot study reported in chapter 6 is a reliable indicator, over the course of a few years you could progress from osteoporosis through osteopenia and into the normal range of bone mineral density, and the appropriate version of each pose will shift accordingly.

You may find that even though your DEXA score is within the normal range, the osteopenia or osteoporosis variation of the pose is the most that you can handle at this point. Follow your own best judgment and do not be discouraged. After all, that version is sufficient to improve bones that are weaker than yours, so it will probably help you as well. Furthermore, just performing that pose at that level may well enable you to progress to the next level in your practice.

Savasana, Corpse Pose, is the last pose in each series. It is a position of total rest after completing any of the three series at any combination of levels. It is a critical part of integrating the gains of the session, and readying yourself for whatever comes your way next.

If you find you're stiff the day after doing these exercises, slow down a little, but keep practicing until that stiffness disappears. Stiffness is normal and will probably fade in a day or two. If you're having trouble doing the poses, consult a teacher or therapist who can find suitable starting postures that work well for you. You may choose to mix the levels in your regimen, with some poses at the easiest level and others at more challenging ones.

How long should you hold a pose? Since bone-forming proteins seem to synthesize quite well after 10 seconds of stimulating pressure, all poses should be held a little longer than that. Try 20 to 30 seconds at first; some may be held up to a minute unless otherwise specified.

Do not feel that if you're at an osteoporosis or osteopenia level that you aren't really doing yoga. Yoga is thousands of years old and has developed in that time to include a vast spectrum of practices. If yoga is that old, so is the teaching of yoga, and so are the elementary poses used to teach it! For the people with osteoporosis or osteopenia, we have excerpted essential elements of the classical poses so that the benefits are considerable there, too. We are not the first to do so; any good teacher knows how to modify poses for specific needs.

In 2007 we surveyed 33,000 yoga therapists and teachers; the results indicated that trying too hard is the main source of the few injuries that do occur in yoga.[1] Remember, the purpose of yoga is to gain control, not lose it. Follow this ancient Chinese advice: "Be not afraid of going slowly, but of standing still."

In spite of its ancient traditional origins, we are advocating yoga from the standpoint of science, not orthodoxy. We have tried to understand the effects of yoga in empirical, objective terms. We have also focused on a few poses, using MRI analyses of their muscular dynamics to relate yoga's effects to the principles of bone growth and morphology. A modern anatomical and biochemical approach might result in more people practicing yoga as an effective medical treatment.

We recognize that there are other ways of doing many of these postures, and that there is nothing sacrosanct about the versions we present.

The yoga therapists and teachers we surveyed found poor alignment to be the second greatest cause of injuries. What we advocate has stood the test of time of two major schools of yoga, Iyengar and Anusara. However, there may well be good and safe alternatives. These differences may be more of style than of substance. The vertebral alignments of the different practitioners from different schools may be almost indistinguishable, provided basic principles are observed.

But that does not mean that just any yoga will do. On the contrary, it suggests that there are something like universal guidelines to correctly do the postures. Earlier we saw that curving the spine forward, as some people might be tempted to do in forward bends, can actually cause fractures. Of all the things to watch for, two deserve special attention: resisting the urge to curve the back in this way, and avoiding falls. That is what the three stages of each pose are about: simple, safe ways of approaching the classical postures.

Special adaptations might be needed for some amputees, stroke victims, and people with particular weaknesses or disabilities. For instance, if you have cervical stenosis, arching the head backward is inadvisable (the

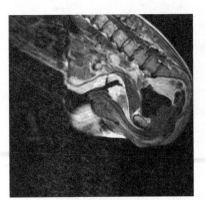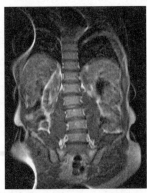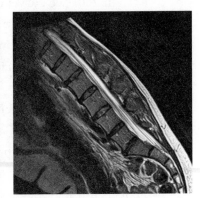

Figure 24. *Though taught by different schools, in different decades, on different continents, with different genders and widely varied years of practice, the substantive differences in the alignment of the lumbar spines here are not great.*

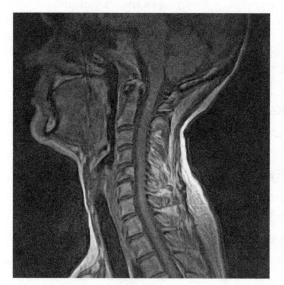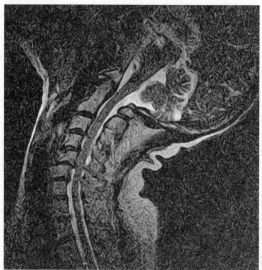

Figure 25. *Neck extension reduces the diameter the already narrow intraspinal canal considerably, producing a spondylolisthesis at the fifth cervical vertebra. (The longer top vertebra is actually the second cervical.) Compare the almost normal, mildly narrowed canal in a neutral position (left) with the dangerously compressed spinal cord that occurs during extension (right). Experienced teachers use extreme caution with extreme extension.*

MRIs in figure 25 illustrate possible dangers). Also, when teaching very young people, it is frequently wiser to focus on the general pose, without fine-tuning, since this may be taken as negative judgment and turn students away from the entire enterprise. It is more helpful for them to do and enjoy doing the yoga than for each refinement to be observed in its totality. A competent teacher/therapist is a valuable source of wisdom and safe practice in these cases.

Absolute and Relative Contraindications

Anything with effects also has side effects; yoga is no exception. For example, a woman with carpal tunnel syndrome should not attempt Downward

Facing Dog, and must be careful with any pose that places much weight on the palm. Common and important precautions are listed with each pose. There are relatively few absolute contraindications—conditions that rule out the pose entirely for you. Unless specifically stated, all the contraindications are relative, meaning that taking into consideration their severity and your ability to adapt, there is probably a way for you to do the pose provided you take the necessary precautions. You need only stay away from the poses to which you have an absolute contraindication.

It may be wise to make a list of any current or recurrent problems you have and check them against the contraindications for the poses. If you find any reason for special care, arrange a suitable adaptation or at least go through the pose's instructions with attentive caution before attempting it. Certainly, if you take a yoga class, tell the instructor about your current list before it starts.

Sometimes a distinction is made between yoga teachers and yoga therapists. There is some practical and theoretical justification for this: Teachers generally have a number of people in front of them when they teach; therapy sessions are most frequently one on one. Teachers generally aim to improve their students' health and enhance joy, while therapists usually set themselves to rid their patients of specific pains or problems. *Yoga for Osteoporosis* may transcend the distinction, since the chief focus is prevention, and teaching is the therapy, practicing is the treatment.

Compliance

In spite of the technological advantage afforded by the DEXA scan and the powerful effects of available medicines, less than 35 percent of the people who are prescribed medicines are actually taking them. In yoga, the rates of continuity are very high. The comparison to medications is not entirely fair, since folks are *told* to take medicine, while many wander into yoga classes of their own volition. However one construes it, yoga is potent (and palatable) medicine.

Some Helpful Technical and Inspirational Points

Props are used in some of these poses, especially in the poses for people with osteoporosis and osteopenia. These props are:

- a bare wall
- a table
- a chair (ideally simple but sturdy folding chairs)
- 3 to 5 blankets
- 2 yoga mats
- 3 blocks or books
- 2 bolsters or cushions
- 2 belts
- 1 small towel

If these items are difficult for you to obtain, be creative in finding household items that serve the same purpose. For example, a strong shoebox may be able to serve as a block. As you progress in the practice, you will need fewer props.

Yoga is a practice that calls upon us to participate holistically. It is not only mechanical exercise for the muscles and joints; it invites an involvement of the intellect and the spirit. One good place to start is to tell yourself that you can do it. Yoga is for everyone, and this book is written to encourage those who might not think they can do yoga because they are unfamiliar with it or they think that they are too stiff.

Yoga practice is an acknowledgment that we are more than our material selves—that our aspirations and deep feelings are also part of what defines us as human beings. We invite you to explore this practice with careful thought and feeling, and to give yourself the solid affirmation that it will help you become stronger, happier, and more liberated. Your body will become an expression of your unique beauty and strength. With practice, your poses will improve, and the effects will carry over into other aspects of your life: better concentration, greater ability to adapt physically and mentally to whatever life brings to you, and deeper self-understanding and acceptance. Yoga offers all of these benefits and more.

Yoga poses are not static positions that we simply hold while waiting for a certain amount of time to pass. In the instructions that follow, you will see many separate actions described in sequence, each of which contributes to the effectiveness of the pose. Each action builds on the one before, and when you remain active in each step of the process, the benefits are considerable. Please read all the instructions over once before actually doing the pose, then try to follow each step as best you can.

Now we will offer some basic technical points that apply to every pose.

The Breath

Be attentive. Actually observing your breath and discovering how to breathe naturally can enhance the poses. Holding the breath blocks awareness and causes fatigue. To begin each pose, expand your body from within on each inhalation. Picture your body actually becoming fuller and lighter inside. This fullness of breath will signal your entire body and mind to be open and receptive. Softly release unnecessary tension with each exhalation. In general, inhale when lifting up or arching your back; exhale when settling into the pose or folding forward. The work of getting into the pose will be easier when supported by awareness of your breathing.

The Foundation

The foundation is the part of the body bearing weight and touching the floor or the chair; it is most often the feet, the hands, or the pelvis. It is important to spread the foundation so that it gives good support. In the feet, this involves identifying and using the four corners of each foot in a balanced way (see figure 26). Press each corner down in the order indicated, and notice how the weight is distributed on your feet. Lift your inner arches while still pressing those four corners down. In addition, stretching the toes instead of contracting them will help with stability and balance.

In the hands use the analogous four corners: the base of the index finger, the inner wrist, the base of the little finger, and the outer wrist.

One good way to set the foundation in the pelvis is with a manual adjustment. Use both hands to adjust each leg in turn. For the left leg, hold the inner thigh with your right hand and the buttock with your left hand as pictured in figure 27. Lean to the right to reduce the weight on the left, and manually revolve the thigh so that the inner edge rolls down. At the same time pull the buttock out and back. Then sit on the left side and adjust the right side. When you are finished you will probably feel your sitting bones more clearly, and be able to lift the spine with more ease. The adjustment is useful for sitting on a chair or the floor.

Parallel Feet

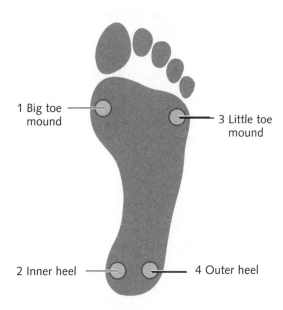

1 Big toe mound

3 Little toe mound

2 Inner heel

4 Outer heel

Figure 26. *Balance your weight on the four corners of each foot for optimal support in all standing poses.*

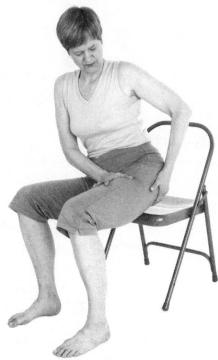

Figure 27. *When sitting, manually widening the pelvis helps to set the foundation for the spine. To widen the pelvis, pull each buttock and upper thigh back and to the side.*

In many poses you will read the instruction to "place the feet parallel" to each other. To achieve parallel feet, draw an imaginary line from the center of your ankle through the center of your second toe. That line should run straight forward and back at all points equidistant to a similar line through the other foot.

The Natural Curves of the Spine When Standing

When observed from the side, the spine has a natural curvature that allows for resilience and freedom of movement. Although there are an infinite number of individual variations to this curvature, there are some general principles.

The lower back and neck are both designed to have a slightly concave shape, to be more hollow at the back. The chest and sacrum will naturally

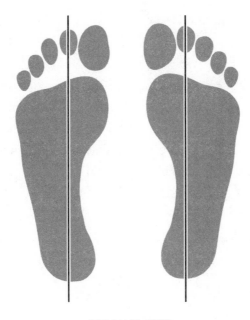

PARALLEL FEET

Figure 28. *The lines from the centers of the ankles to the second toes are facing straight forward and are parallel.*

have a more convex, rounded shape toward the back. Ideally the curves are moderate and not exaggerated.

To adjust and stabilize the lower back, first move the tops of the thigh bones back, which creates more lumbar arch, then curl the tailbone down to lengthen the spine. Avoid pushing the thighs forward as the tailbone moves down and in.

To align the middle back, move the sides of the waistline back to prevent a swayback. Then lift the front chest up with support from the shoulder blades in back. This reduces the forward curve of the thoracic spine, typical of slumped posture.

For the neck and head, tip your chin up just a bit to create the concave curve of the neck, then reach up with the back of the head to create length in the neck. Ideally the head is neither jutting forward nor pulling excessively back, but balanced directly over the axis of the spine.

Your goal when aligning the spine is to have a balance of strength and flexibility in the back and front of the spine. Modern life is quite sedentary, encouraging a forward-bending posture of the spine—longer in the back, shorter in the front. This posture sets the stage for increased fracture risk. When practicing forward bends especially, move your whole back forward from as low down in the spine as possible. Tilt the pelvis forward from the hips, not the waist. This will minimize any rounding of the spine. Aligning your back this way may not be easy at first due to tightness in your legs, but it is crucial for the safety and effectiveness of the poses.

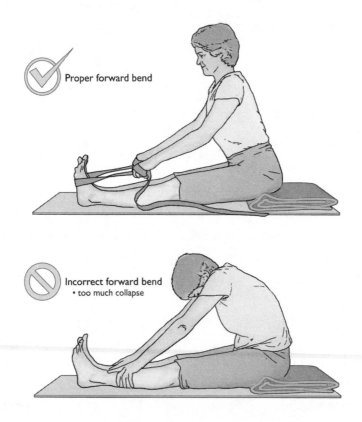

Proper forward bend

Incorrect forward bend
• too much collapse

CORRECT AND INCORRECT FORWARD BEND:
NOTE THE SHAPE OF THE SPINE

Figure 29. *Bend forward from the hips, not from the waist, to maximize the benefits of these poses and to avoid vertebral fractures.*

Back-bending yoga poses stimulate the vertebral bodies, lengthen the front of the spine, and balance pressure on the disks. The poses that arch your back contribute to balance in another way as well: while forward bends produce calm, backbends are exhilarating.

The Balance of Opposites

If you are doing yoga for the first time, you may wonder why the pose instructions include actions that are opposite. We may instruct you to press down and then reach up, or turn in and then turn out, for example. The goal is to create a stable and balanced pressure on the bones, which makes the poses safer and more effective. Below is an introduction to some of these pairs of opposite actions.

Pulling In and Reaching Out

The benefits of yoga for osteoporosis derive from the pull of muscle on bone. Yoga is not a relaxed practice in which the body simply folds into a shape and drapes there with great ease. We need to engage a muscular strength that contracts and brings the different parts of the body toward the center by pulling on the bones. For example, a common instruction will be to retract the arms into the shoulder sockets.

The opposite action, extending out from the center, also stimulates the bones and prevents excessive compression of the joints. In each pose we aim for a balance between contraction and expansion. Think of the opposition of forces that occurs when you put on a glove. With one hand you pull the glove in over your hand, while the other hand pushes forward into the glove. The balance of both actions, inward pull and outward push, accomplishes that task and is our goal.

Rooting Down and Extending Upward

Another example in which we employ movement in opposite directions simultaneously is when we create a strong foundation and then reach up from it. "Rooting" into the foundation means actively pressing down, a movement that will initiate a natural lift in the rest of the body. For instance, when sitting, if you reach your sitting bones down and back, your lower back will naturally arch slightly and rise up. Like the feeling of rebound when you are about to jump, the downward motion of your legs gives the needed push-off for upward momentum. When airborne in a jump the body is extending both up and down, and we do this same kind of two-directional expansion in yoga poses.

Inward and Outward Rotation of the Legs and Arms

The limbs are endowed with a wide range of motion for the myriad types of activities asked of them. We have a complex array of muscles to use for movements, and good alignment entails coordinating them so the work is properly shared. You will notice instructions to turn the legs or arms inward and then outward; doing both will secure the arm or leg in its socket for good stability and apply dynamic pressure to the bones involved.

The Knees

In most poses, align each kneecap to face the same direction as the second toe of that same leg. If this is not easy, work toward it gradually. This alignment protects the knee from dangerous torque.

How to Measure Your Stance

In many standing poses, the feet are wide apart. The distance between your feet will vary with your height, your proportions, and your flexibility. Some instructions for standing poses will ask you to start with your feet wide enough apart to situate your wrists above your ankles when you stretch your arms horizontally. If that feels too wide or unstable, adjust it until you feel right. The stance should allow for both freedom (the hips are generally more moveable with a wider stance) and stability.

Tadasana

Tadasana, Mountain Pose, is referenced occasionally in the text as a pose for transitioning or resting between the right and left sides of a pose, or between one pose and the next. In Tadasana we stand tall with inner and outer strength, with simplicity and dignity. All of the alignments described above can be learned in Tadasana, making it a foundational pose. Use it whenever you need a moment to renew your focus and realign yourself.

Practicing with Written Instructions

To avoid the awkwardness of doing a yoga pose while holding a book in your hands, we recommend the following: Read the instructions for the pose over several times to understand the full extent of what you'll do. Then go over it with frequent reference to the book for a few days, after which you and your body will probably remember what to do. You can also have a friend or teacher read the instructions aloud, or tape-record yourself reading them. Periodically read over the instructions to check that you have included each part of each pose. The descriptions of the alignment and actions of each pose are crucial to safety and effectiveness, so don't rush to get to the final shape.

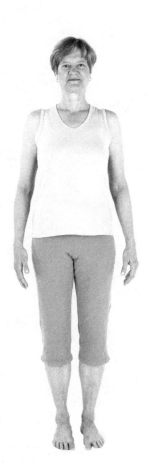

Every Pose Is a Full-Body Pose

Each pose will probably bring your focus to one or two areas of the body, due to the strength or stretching it requires. In a standing pose you might feel your legs more; in a sitting pose your spine or

Figure 30. *Tadasana, the Mountain Pose*

your shoulders might be the center of your attention. We invite you to open your awareness to your whole body in every pose. Maximize your work and your time by enlivening yourself fully, rather just doing the bare minimum. Your work will not go to waste, and the therapeutic effects for osteoporosis and everything else will grow. Notice the details, but also the overall dynamics, the form and feeling of the poses. Make them your own. Be confident that you will receive the therapeutic benefits of yoga practice and your skills will improve over time.

Chapter 9

Poses That Focus on Bone Strength

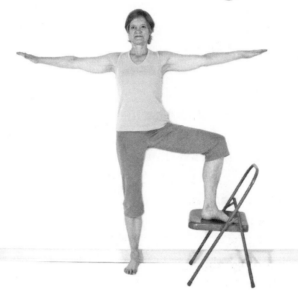

I. VRKSASANA Tree Pose

Purpose: To strengthen the legs and hips, improve balance without risk, and improve posture and focus.

Contraindications: Severe rotator cuff injury, imbalance.

Props: A wall and a chair.

Avoiding pitfalls: Use two opposite actions to establish balance: a strong pull of all the muscles onto the bones, and a corresponding outward expansion from the center of your body out through your arms and legs. Too much or too little effort will increase the challenge of balancing.

OSTEOPOROSIS VARIATION

1. Place a chair near a wall, facing to the side.
2. Stand a few inches from the wall with the right side of your body alongside the back of the chair. Rest your right hand lightly on the chair.
3. Position your feet facing straight forward and parallel. Spread your toes.
4. Root down through the four corners of the feet and lift your inner arches up.
5. From the feet, stretch your legs all the way up to the pelvis, using a strong squeezing action in the muscles just above your knees.
6. Pull back through the tops of your thighs and widen your sitting bones. (Leaning forward a little with your upper body makes this easier.)

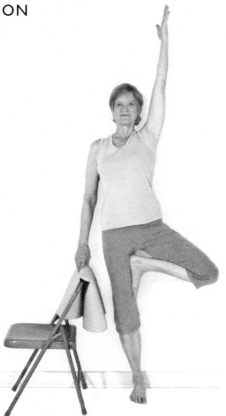

7. Lengthen the back of your pelvis down and lift your abdomen up. As you do this, center your pelvis and spine vertically over your thighs.
8. Pick up your left foot and place the sole of the foot on the inner edge of your right leg as high as you can toward the top of the leg, toes pointing down. Your left knee will face to the side at a diagonal.
9. Push the left foot and right inner leg against each other for stability.
10. Repeat the actions of taking the top thighs back and pulling the abdomen up, to maintain good balance over the standing leg.
11. Using the chair and the wall behind you for balance if you need to, stretch the left arm out to the side or all the way up.

12. Intensely stretch out from the core of your pelvis in all directions, out through your arms, legs, and torso. Embody the strength and dignity of a great tall tree. Continue with full breaths.

13. Hold the pose for as long as you safely can maintain the actions, then bring the left foot down and rest on two feet, sitting down if you need to.

14. Repeat on the second side.

15. Stand on both legs and take several breaths to rest.

Note: If needed for stability, the lifted foot can be placed on a chair, and the arms stretched straight to the side.

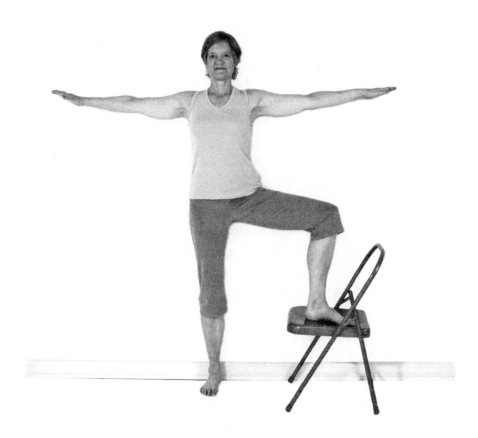

OSTEOPENIA VARIATION

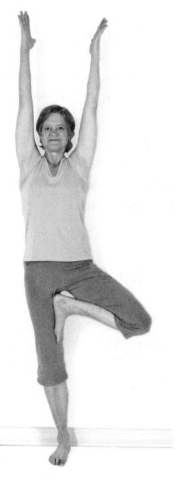

1. Stand with your back a few inches from the wall.
2. Position your feet facing straight forward and parallel. Spread your toes.
3. Root down through the four corners of the feet and lift your inner arches up.
4. From the feet, stretch your legs all the way up to the pelvis, using a strong squeezing action in the muscles just above your knees.
5. Pull back through the tops of your thighs and widen your sitting bones. (Leaning forward a little with your upper body makes this easier.)
6. Lengthen the back of your pelvis down and lift your abdomen up. As you do this, align your pelvis and spine vertically over your thighs.
7. Pick up your left foot and place the sole of the foot on the inner edge of your right leg as high as you can toward the top of the leg, toes pointing down. Turn your left knee to the side as much as possible without turning your pelvis.
8. Push the left foot and right inner leg against each other for stability.
9. Redo the actions of taking the thighs back and pulling the abdomen up to maintain good balance over the standing leg.
10. Look straight ahead, finding a place across the room to focus on. This will help you to balance.
11. Take a big inhalation and stretch your arms out to the side and up as far as you can toward vertical. Touch the wall gently if you need to.
12. Intensely stretch out from the core of your pelvis in all directions, out

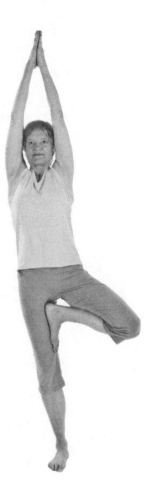

through your arms, down through your legs, and up through your torso. Embody the strength and dignity of a great tall tree.

13. Hold the pose for as long as you can maintain the actions, then bring the left foot down and rest on two feet.

14. Stand on both legs and take several breaths to rest.

15. Repeat on the second side.

16. Stand on both legs and take several breaths to rest.

PREVENTION VARIATION

1. Stand with your feet together and spread your toes.

2. Root down through the four corners of the feet and lift your inner arches up.

3. From the feet, stretch your legs all the way up to the pelvis, using a strong squeezing action in the muscles just above your knees.

4. Pull back through the tops of your thighs and widen your sitting bones. (Leaning forward a little with your upper body makes this easier.)

5. Lengthen the back of your pelvis down and lift your abdomen up. As you do this, align your pelvis and spine vertically over your thighs.

6. Bring your left foot up to the top of the inner right thigh, with the toes pointing down. Press the right thigh and left foot against each other strongly for stability. Bring the left knee to the side as much as possible without turning your pelvis.

7. Redo the actions of taking the thighs back and pulling the abdomen up to maintain good balance of the pelvis over the standing leg.

8. Look straight ahead. Find a place across the room on which to focus. This will help you to balance.

9. Take a full inhalation and stretch your arms out to the side and up as

far as you can toward vertical. You may join your palms together or keep the arms straight up near your ears. Pull your shoulders back.

10. Intensely stretch out from the core of your pelvis in all directions: out through your arms, down through your legs, and up through your torso. Embody the strength and dignity of a great tall tree.

11. Continue will full breaths, stretching especially through the thumbs.

12. Hold the pose for as long as you can maintain the actions, then bring the left foot down and rest on two feet.

13. Repeat on the second side.

14. Stand on both legs and take several breaths to rest.

2. UTKATASANA   Chair Pose

Purpose: To stress the entire pelvis and all posterior portions of the spine's vertebrae, and to strengthen the quadriceps. To build inner and outer strength.

Contraindications: Imbalance, acromioclavicular subluxation, rotator

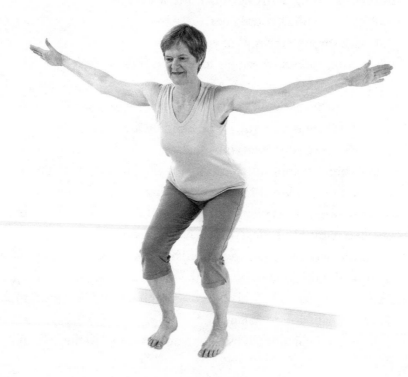

cuff tear, profound weakness, anterior cruciate tear grades III–IV, chondromalacia patellae, plantar fasciitis.

Props: A yoga mat and a wall (osteoporosis variation).

Avoiding pitfalls: Take care to align the knees—track the kneecaps straight forward over the second toes. Align the lower back: neither too arched nor too curved forward.

OSTEOPOROSIS VARIATION

1. Stand on your mat facing away from a wall and adjust the distance so that when you bend your knees and flex your hips, your buttocks rest against the wall. Set your feet hip-width apart and parallel.
2. Inhaling, bend your knees, reach your hips back to the wall, and raise your arms to horizontal in one vigorous movement.
3. Lift your toes, especially the fourth and fifth, and root the heels down.
4. Isometrically push your thighs apart while still tracking the kneecaps straight forward over the second and third toes.
5. As your hips draw back, allow your lower back to arch, producing a deep fold in your hips.
6. Lift the lower abdomen up to support the lower back and reduce the lumbar arch.
7. Breathe calmly and maintain the position for as long as you can.
8. Inhale as you come back up. Exhaling, lower your arms.

OSTEOPENIA VARIATION

1. Stand on your mat with your feet hip-width apart and parallel.
2. Inhaling, bend your knees, reach your hips back and apart, and raise your arms to the sides in one vigorous movement. Bring your arms above shoulder height if possible, with your palms forward. The arms stretch up at a diagonal.
3. Lift your toes, especially the fourth and fifth, and root the heels down.
4. Isometrically push your thighs apart while still tracking the kneecaps straight forward over the second and third toes.

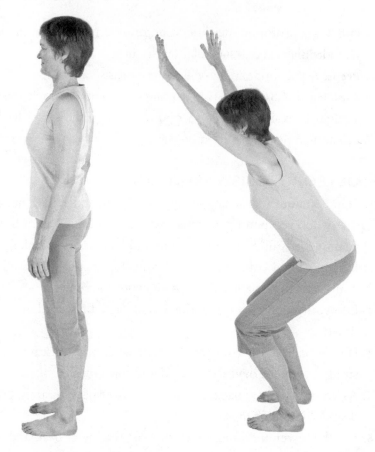

5. As your hips draw back, allow your lower back to arch, producing a deep fold in your hips.
6. Lift the lower abdomen up to support the lower back and lessen the lumbar arch.
7. Breathe calmly and maintain the position for as long as you can.
8. Inhale to come back up. Exhale as you lower your arms.

PREVENTION VARIATION
1. Stand on your mat with your feet hip-width apart and parallel.
2. Inhale, bend your knees, reach your hips back and apart, and sweep your arms out to the sides until your upper arms are near your ears, all in one vigorous movement.

3. Pull back through the upper arms as you turn your palms toward each other and stretch the arms fully.

4. Lift your toes, especially the fourth and fifth, and root the heels down.

5. Isometrically push your thighs apart while still tracking the kneecaps straight forward over the second and third toes.

6. As your hips draw back, allow your lower back to arch, producing a deep fold in your hips.

7. Lift the lower abdomen up to support the lower back and lessen the lumbar curve.

8. Breathe calmly and maintain the position for as long as you can.

9. Inhale to come back up. Exhale as you lower your arms.

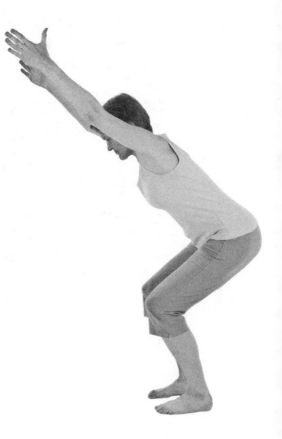

3. UTTHITA TRIKONASANA   Triangle Pose

Purpose: To stress the greater trochanters, put strong torque pressure on the anterior lumbar and posterior thoracic vertebra and the pubic rami, to build stamina, focus, and balance.

Contraindications: Newly herniated disc, advanced hip arthritis, pubic fracture, Achilles tendonitis, ligamentous knee injuries, knee arthritis.

Props: A yoga mat, along with a wall, chair, or block for some variations.

Avoiding pitfalls: The wider your stance, the more freedom you'll have in the hips, but don't go so wide as to lose stability. The knees may want to bend and the upper body tends to shift forward. Keep your legs straight, your leg muscles firm, and your torso lined up directly above your front leg.

OSTEOPOROSIS VARIATION

1. Place your yoga mat next to a wall. Place the chair next to the wall, facing toward you, near the front of your mat.
2. Stand with your back to the wall. Step your feet apart so that your ankles line up under your wrists when your arms stretch to the sides. Turn the right foot and leg parallel to the wall, but face your torso straight out from the wall. Your right toes will be just under the chair. Internally rotate the left foot 30 degrees toward the right. Align your right heel with the arch of your left foot.
3. With your arms remaining outstretched, incline your torso to the right without bending it. Your hips will shift to the left. Rest your right hand on the chair seat, and stretch your left hand out to the side.

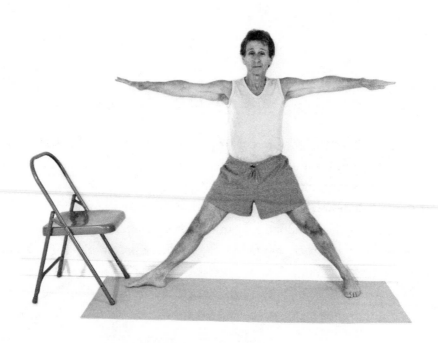

4. Inhale, firm your legs to keep them straight, and widen your sitting bones. Move the inner thighs back and apart.

5. Curl your tailbone down toward the left heel. Lift your abdomen up.

6. Lengthen out through the spine. Exhale and shift your hips more to the left. Extend your torso out over your right leg, bending at the hips, not the waist. The stretch occurs in the back of the right leg and the left side of the pelvis.

7. Distribute your weight more or less equally on both feet.

8. Keep both sides of the torso long and parallel with a full stretch from your pelvis to the crown of your head. Avoid collapsing down by extending the spine horizontally.

9. If you are unsteady, lean your right hip and one or both shoulders lightly against the wall.

10. Roll your left shoulder, left ribs, and left waist back and up, remaining steady in your legs. Face straight forward, toward the middle of the room.

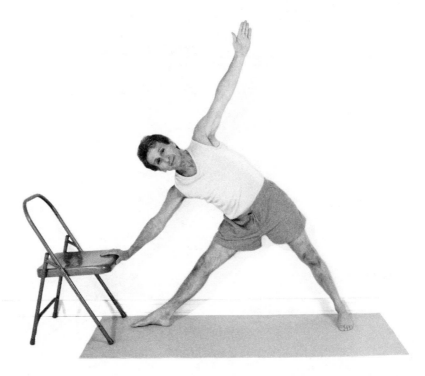

11. Radiate energy out through all your limbs and your spine. Stretch side to side as well as head to tail.

12. Inhale as you come back up.

13. Repeat on the second side. You can stand in Tadasana (see page 93) between sides if you wish.

OSTEOPENIA VARIATION

1. Place your yoga mat along a wall, and a block near the end of your mat on the right side.

2. Stand with your back to the wall but not touching it, and step your feet apart so that your ankles line up under your wrists when your arms stretch to the sides. Place your right foot next to the block, and turn the foot and leg parallel to the wall but aim your torso straight out from the wall. Internally rotate your left foot 30 degrees toward the right. Align your right heel with the arch of your left foot.

3. With your arms remaining outstretched, incline your torso to the

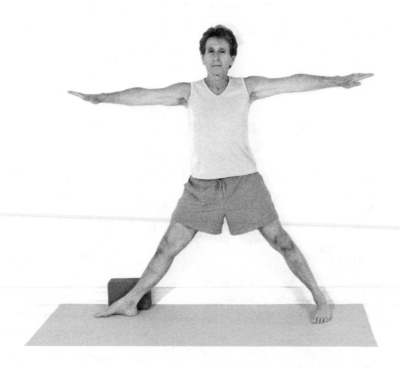

right without bending it. Your hips will shift to the left. Rest your right hand on the block, left hand on your waist.

4. Inhale, firm your legs to keep them straight, and widen your sitting bones, moving the inner thighs back and apart.

5. Curl your tailbone diagonally down toward the left heel and lift your abdomen up.

6. Lengthen out through the spine. Exhale and shift your hips more to the left. Extend your torso out over your right leg, bending at the hips, not the waist. The stretch occurs in the back of the right leg and the left side of the pelvis.

7. Distribute your weight more or less equally on both feet.

8. Keep both sides of the torso long and parallel with a full stretch from your pelvis to the crown of your head. Avoid collapsing down by extending the spine horizontally.

9. If you are unsteady, lean your right hip and one or both shoulders lightly against the wall.

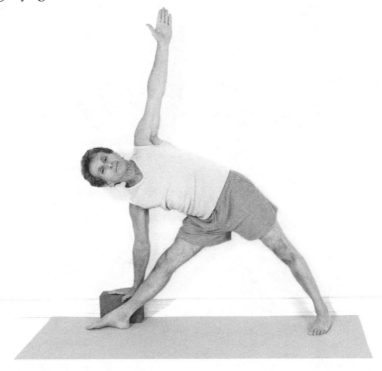

10. Roll your left shoulder, left ribs, and left waist back and up, remaining steady in your legs. Stretch your left arm straight up toward the ceiling. Face straight forward, toward the middle of the room.

11. Breathing fully, radiate energy out through all your limbs and your spine. Stretch side to side as well as head to tail.

12. Inhale as you come back up.

13. Repeat on the second side. You can stand in Tadasana (see page 93) between sides if you wish.

PREVENTION VARIATION

1. Step your feet apart so that your ankles line up under your wrists when your arms stretch to the sides. Turn your right foot and leg 90 degrees to the right, but do not turn your torso. Internally rotate your left foot 30 degrees toward the right. Align your right heel with the arch of your left foot.

2. Inhale and stretch your arms firmly, pulling your shoulder blades toward your spine.

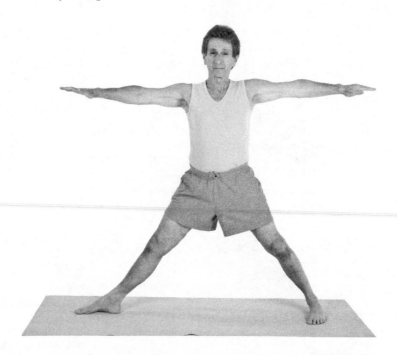

3. Exhale and incline your torso to the right without bending or turning it. Your hips will shift to the left. Touch the floor on the outside of your right foot with your fingertips, or place your hand over your ankle. Rest your left hand on your waist.

4. Inhale, firm your legs to keep them straight, and widen your sitting bones, moving the inner thighs back and apart.

5. Curl your tailbone diagonally down toward your left heel and lift your abdomen up.

6. Lengthen out through the spine. Exhale and shift your hips more to the left. Extend your torso out over your right leg, bending at the hips, not the waist. The stretch occurs in the back of the right leg and the left side of the pelvis.

7. Distribute your weight more or less equally on both feet.

8. Keep both sides of the torso long and parallel with a full stretch from your pelvis to the crown of your head. Avoid collapsing down by extending the spine horizontally.

9. Roll your left shoulder, left ribs, and left waist back and up, remaining

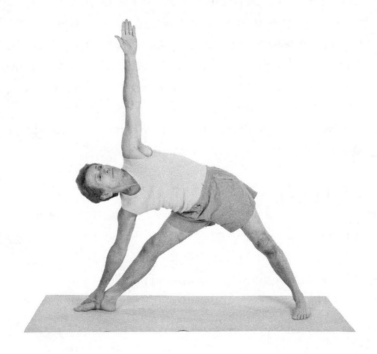

steady in your legs. Stretch your left arm straight up toward the ceiling. Turn your head to look up at your left hand.

11. Breathing fully, radiate energy out through all your limbs and your spine. Stretch side to side as well as head to tail.

12. Inhale as you come back up.

13. Repeat on the second side. You can stand in Tadasana (see page 93) between sides if you wish.

4. ADHO MUKHA SVANASANA
Downward Facing Dog

Purpose: To stress the posterior thigh and shin bones, calcaneus, inner humerus, forearm bones, wrists, shoulder blades, lower anterior ribs, and posterior elements of all vertebrae. This is a particularly invigorating pose.

Contraindications: Acromioclavicular dysfunction, rotator cuff tear, thoracic outlet syndrome, spondylolisthesis, Dupuytren's contractures, carpal tunnel syndrome, Achilles tendon tear.

Props: A yoga mat, wall, and chair.

Avoiding pitfalls: Retract the shoulder blades firmly onto the back ribs; don't let the upper arms sag downward. Roll the inner arms upward toward the ceiling to maintain the proper rotation of the upper arms. This will help to firm your elbows in toward the midline, providing stability in the pose. Keep the knees bent if you are stiff, in order to be able to tilt the pelvis and lengthen the spine.

OSTEOPOROSIS VARIATION

1. Place your yoga mat next to a wall. Stand 12 to 14 inches from the wall and place your hands on the wall above eye level, index fingers pointing up and the arms shoulder-width apart.

2. Place your feet hip-width apart and parallel.

3. Straighten your arms and move your chest a little toward the wall.

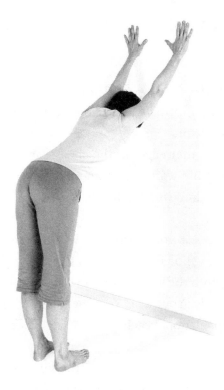

4. Move your upper arms more securely back into the shoulder joints.

5. Keep your elbows straight and your upper arms light but active.

6. Bend forward through your trunk until there is one long diagonal line from hands to hips. You can step back as needed. Do not round your back.

7. Stretch back with your sitting bones and separate them, which will make an arch in your lower back.

8. Draw in your belly and lengthen the tailbone back.

9. Let the thoracic spine soften downward without collapsing your arms.

10. If your hamstrings allow, do the pose with straight legs. If your hamstrings are tight, your knees can be bent slightly in order to allow the pelvis to tilt properly. Find the degree of effort in extending yourself that feels good, using your breath.

11. After several breaths, come back up as you inhale and step toward the wall.

OSTEOPENIA VARIATION

1. Place a chair against the wall, facing out toward you. Place your mat in front of the chair.
2. Hold the front outer edges of the chair seat and walk your feet back, feet remaining hip-width apart and parallel. How far you step back will vary according to your flexibility; go as far as you can without losing stability.
3. Bend your knees as you reach your hips back to stretch the spine and arms in one long line from hands to hips.
4. Breathe fully into the sides of the rib cage and maintain strength in all parts of the body. Your head stays between your arms.
5. With each inhalation, reach your sitting bones up, back and apart. Make space.
6. With each exhalation, elongate all the lines of the pose (legs, arms, spine). Expand out strongly from the inside.
7. Stretch your legs straight if you can, without curling the back of the pelvis down. You can step back farther, and your heels can be off the floor.
8. To come out of the pose, walk toward the chair and stand up.

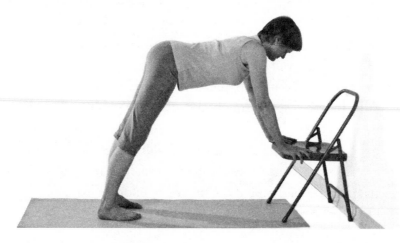

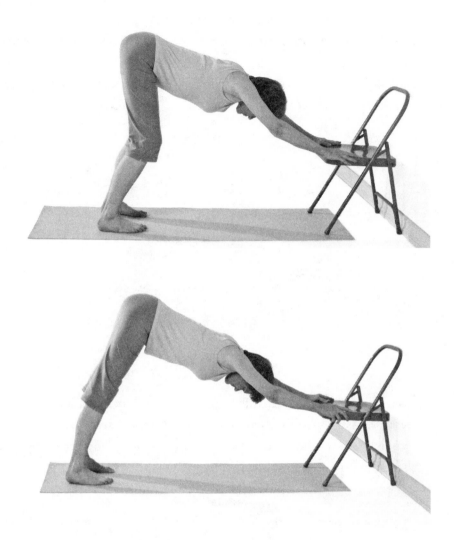

PREVENTION VARIATION

1. Come down onto your hands and knees on your mat. Walk your knees back a bit farther than your hips. Place your hands at the front of the mat, shoulder-width apart, fingers separated, index fingers pointing forward.

2. Firm your arm muscles, press your fingers down, and soften your chest down over the tops of the arms so that the arms connect solidly into the shoulder sockets.

3. Draw your shoulder blades in toward your spine.

4. Tuck your toes under and make space in the sides and front of your entire torso.

5. Inhale and lift up your knees and hips, elevating the sitting bones back, up and apart.

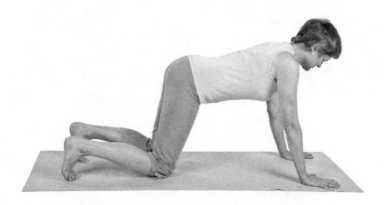

6. As you exhale, stretch fully through your arms and spine, pulling your legs back still farther. If your hamstrings are very tight, bend your knees to allow your pelvis to tilt properly. Gradually work to straighten your knees.

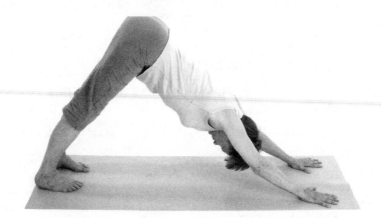

7. Create a slight concavity in the lumbar and thoracic spine by reaching upward with the sitting bones.

8. As you become more flexible, you will be able to pull the thighs back with straight knees, and eventually lower your heels.

9. Once you have created the full pose, sensitively extend through all parts of the body, from the core to the periphery. Charge your body with strength.

10. To release, bring your knees to the floor.

5. BHUJANGASANA AND URDHVA MUKHA SVANASANA   Prone Backbends

Purpose: To stimulate the posterior elements of the entire spine, shoulder joint, arms and wrists.

Contraindications: Fused ankylosing spondylitis, Arnold-Chiari syndrome, bridging spondylitis, cervical spinal stenosis, spondylolisthesis, carpal tunnel syndrome.

Props: A yoga mat and a blanket.

Avoiding pitfalls: Keep your shoulders back and the sides of your body long. Don't overuse your arms. If you get up into the pose and find your shoulders around your ears and your chest collapsed, come down and start over. This pose is about expanding from the inside and supporting yourself with the muscles of your spine, more than the muscles in your arms.

OSTEOPOROSIS VARIATION

1. Lie on your stomach with a blanket under you for comfort.

2. Lift one leg up an inch and lengthen it away from the pelvis. Repeat with the other leg. This creates a good length in the lower back.

3. Briefly turn the fronts of your legs in toward the midline, so that the heels, thighs, and pelvis widen in the back.

4. Pull your tailbone toward your heels and toward the floor. This stabilizes your lower back, enabling you to stretch forward more strongly.

The legs will rotate back to center; the heels and backs of the knees will face straight up.

5. Lift yourself up onto your forearms briefly to pull your upper body forward, away from your legs.

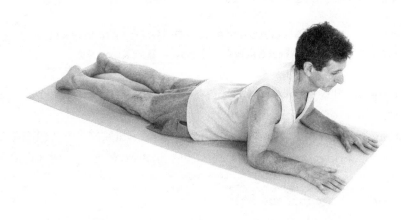

6. Lie back down and place your hands a few inches away from the sides of your chest, fingers pointing outward a bit, forehead on the floor.

7. Lift your shoulders away from the floor, keeping them square across.

8. Inhale and lengthen your whole torso forward. Expand from the inside.

9. Contract your upper back muscles and move the shoulder blades in toward the spine. Curl your head and chest upward and keep your shoulders back.

10. Carefully press down to lift more, but keep your arms bent and the upper arms and shoulders back.

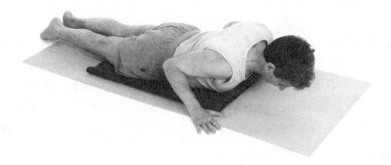

11. Use your breath to expand forward from inside, lengthening the sides of the body.
12. Stay up for several breaths, then soften and release down.

OSTEOPENIA VARIATION

Follow preparation steps 1–10 in the osteoporosis variation.

11. Come up as high as you can, using your breath to expand forward from the inside.
12. Press the hands down through their four corners and pull up through the upper arms, creating length through the sides of the ribs. Rise up with confidence.
13. Stay up for several breaths, then soften and release down.

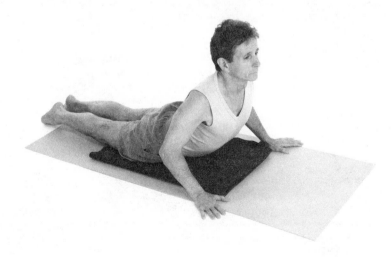

PREVENTION VARIATION

Follow steps 1–11 above in the osteoporosis variation.

12. Pull your upper body forward on the mat until your chest emerges in front of your upper arms and your hands are under your shoulders.

13. Strongly push down through your hands, curl your shoulders back, and arch your upper back. Your pelvis will rise off the floor as you straighten your arms, but you can leave your knees and lower legs in contact with the floor.

14. Keep the back of the pelvis long as you rise up from the inside and widen the front of your chest. Reach back through your legs.

15. To do a stronger pose, lift your pelvis off the floor as you straighten your arms.

16. Stretch back strongly through your legs with only the tops of your feet touching the floor.

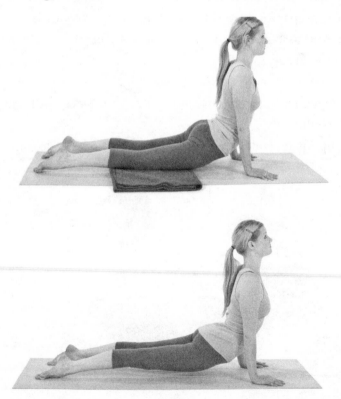

17. Arch your head back and look up.

18. Stay up for several breaths, then soften and release down.

---

6. SETU BANDHASANA   Supine Backbend

Purpose: To stimulate the posterior elements of the entire spine, raising anterior and posterior pressures at the hips, shoulders, and wrists, and flexion pressure on the knees, ankles, and elbows, augmenting gravitational forces. The pose also strengthens the muscles that perform these actions.

Contraindications: (absolute) Arnold-Chiari malformations; (relative) sacroiliac joint derangement, scoliosis, facet syndrome, spinal stenosis, spondylolisthesis, spondylolysis.

Props: A yoga mat, a blanket, a belt, and a block.

Avoiding pitfalls: Keep the legs and feet parallel. Relax your neck, throat, and jaw as you breathe. Avoid squeezing the buttocks too tightly or pulling the arms toward the feet.

OSTEOPOROSIS VARIATION

1. Lie on your back with the tops of your shoulders on the top edge of the folded blanket, your head on the mat. Bend your knees, and place your feet hip-width apart and parallel, about 6 to 8 inches from your hips.

2. Place your arms alongside your body, palms facing up. Take a few breaths, inflate your inner body, and soften any shoulder tension.

3. Inhale and curl your sitting bones down and apart to ensure that the pelvis stays wide.

4. Exhale and firm your abdominal muscles.

5. Lift your hips and chest as you inhale, and place the block under your pelvis. You can choose the orientation of the block: flatter, a bit higher, or highest, according to your ability to extend. Bend your elbows 90 degrees. Point your fingers up toward the ceiling.

6. Once the weight of your lower body is supported on the block, tuck

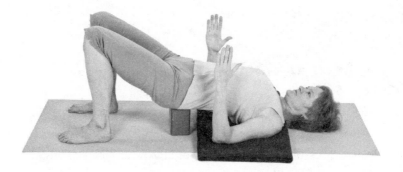

each shoulder under so that the tops of your shoulders are on the blanket.

7. Point your knees straight forward, then lift and extend your tailbone toward your knees.

8. As you inhale, lift your hips off the block, taking care to engage the buttock muscles without squeezing them together too tightly. Lengthen your buttocks toward your knees.

9. Press your shoulders toward the floor by contracting the muscles between your shoulder blades.

10. Hold these two actions—shoulders pressing down, pelvis pressing up—as long as you can. Breathe smoothly.

11. This pose stimulates the lungs as it strengthens the shoulder and back muscles.

12. To come out of the pose, remove the block and lie flat on the floor.

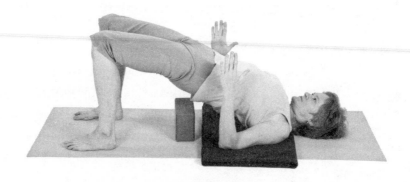

OSTEOPENIA VARIATION

In this variation, resistance against the belt provides increased stimulus to the shoulders and arms.

1. Lie on your back with the tops of your shoulders on the top edge of the folded blanket, your head on the mat. Bend your knees, and place your feet hip-width apart and parallel, about 6 to 8 inches from your hips.

2. Prepare the belt by making a loop that is 10 to 12 inches wide. Put one wrist inside the loop.

3. Place your arms flat alongside your body, palms facing up or in toward the center. Take a few breaths, inflate your chest, and soften any shoulder tension.

4. Inhale and curl your sitting bones down and apart to ensure that the pelvis stays wide.

5. Exhale, firm your abdominal muscles, and pull your arms into the shoulder sockets.

6. Lift your hips and chest as you inhale. Tuck each shoulder under toward the spine so that the tops of your shoulders are on the blanket.

7. Place the second wrist inside the belt loop behind your back, palms facing inward.

8. Point your knees straight forward, then lift and extend your tailbone toward your knees.

9. As you inhale, lift your hips higher, taking care to contract the buttock muscles without squeezing them together too tightly. Lengthen the buttocks toward your knees.

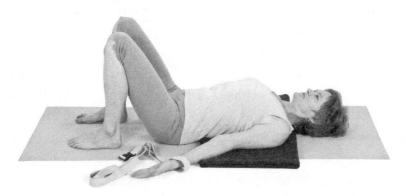

10. Push out against the belt with your arms while pressing them down onto the floor.

11. Continue these two actions—arms pushing down and out, pelvis pressing up—for as long as you can, breathing smoothly. Build your inner strength.

12. To come out of the pose, remove the belt and lie flat on the floor.

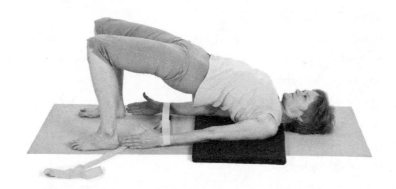

PREVENTION VARIATION

1. Lie on your back, bend your knees, and place your feet hip-width apart and parallel, about 6 to 8 inches from your hips.

2. Place your arms alongside your body, palms facing up. Take a few breaths, inflate your inner body, and soften any shoulder tension.

3. Inhale and curl your sitting bones down and apart to ensure that the pelvis stays wide.

4. Exhale, firm your abdominal muscles, and pull your arms into your shoulder sockets.

5. Lift your hips and chest as you inhale. Tuck each shoulder under toward the spine so that the tops of your shoulders are on the mat.

6. Interlace your fingers behind you, but separate the wrists. Press the arms down into the floor to propel your torso upward.

7. Point your knees straight forward, then lift and extend your tailbone toward your knees.

8. Lengthen the buttocks away from your waist without squeezing them tightly.

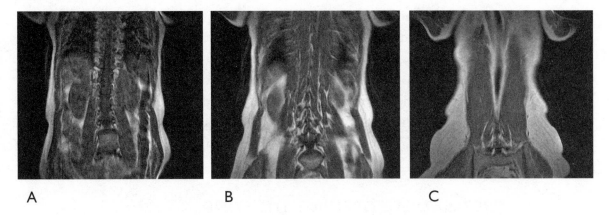

A	B	C

Figure 31. *In back bends, muscles such as the iliopsoas (left), paraspinal muscles (center), and quadratus lumborum (right) pull against and thus stimulate the lumbar vertebral bodies from the front (A) and back (B), indirectly from the sides through the lower ribs (C), and at many angles between (B).*

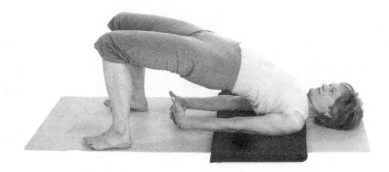

9. Stretch the sides and the center of the body down from your throat out through the legs, unfolding your own power. Breathe smoothly.
10. Exhale softly as you come down.

7. URDHVA DHANURASANA   Upward Bow

This pose is challenging—and fantastic—and is presented here for prevention only. The guidance of an experienced teacher is highly recommended for all variations of this pose. Its strong actions provide valuable stimulus to the bones, but it is not for beginners or those who are stiff or weak.

Purpose: To stimulate the posterior elements for the entire spine and direct extension pressures to the hips, all with the isometric action of opposing muscle groups.

Contraindications: (absolute) Arnold-Chiari malformations, (relative) sacroiliac joint derangement, scoliosis, facet syndrome, spinal stenosis, spondylolisthesis, spondylolysis, cerebrovascular disease.

Props: A folding chair, a wall, two blankets, and two bolsters or cushions.

PREPARATION: OPENING THE SPINE

Avoiding pitfalls: Adjust your position in the chair relative to your height. Taller people will sit farther into the chair in the beginning. Take care to lengthen your back as you arch into the full pose.

1. Place your chair about 2 feet from a wall. Place a folded blanket on the seat.
2. Place the bolster and an extra folded blanket in front of the chair.
3. Sit facing backward in the chair, on the edge of the blanket, your legs threaded beneath the backrest.
4. Manually widen your sitting bones and upper thighs (see pages 87–88).
5. Firm and lift your abdominal muscles.
6. Hold the sides of the backrest with your hands.

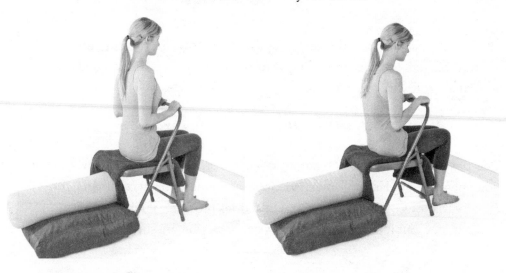

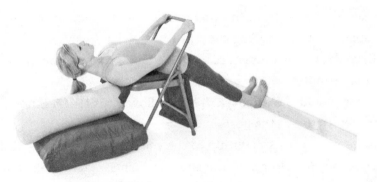

7. Inhaling, lift up your back ribs and bow forward, rounding your spine slightly. This preparatory action prevents compression in the low back.

8. Press your feet against the wall. Exhale and start to lean back, still rounding your back to create length, until your upper back reaches the front edge of the chair. Slide your hips farther into the chair if you need to. Aim to place your upper back (the area between the shoulder blades) at the edge of the chair.

9. Once your back is on the chair but before your shoulders and neck arch more deeply, firm your shoulder blades onto your back and lift your chest up.

10. Move the sides of your neck back and up to lengthen the neck before arching it.

11. Exhaling, arch your shoulders and head back over the front edge of the chair. Rest your head on the bolster and extra blanket, or let it hang if this is comfortable. Your hands can stay on the backrest, and even push lightly to increase the opening of your chest.

12. Push into the wall with your feet and straighten your legs. The chair

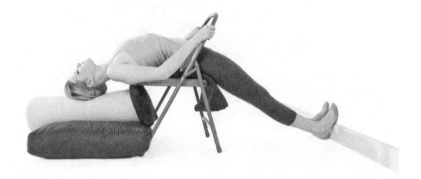

may slide away from the wall a little. Use the action of your legs to support your expanding chest as you arch backward.

13. Extend through your entire body. Let inside and outside merge as you breathe fully.

14. If you would like a deeper stretch, follow steps 15–17. If not, proceed to step 18 to exit the pose.

15. Raise your arms straight up to the ceiling. With the tops of the arm bones staying close into the shoulder joints, extend your arms back and attempt to touch the floor behind your head.

16. Extend your body fully from your feet to the crown of your head and your fingertips. Let inside and outside merge as you breathe fully.

17. To prepare to come up, bring your hands onto the backrest.

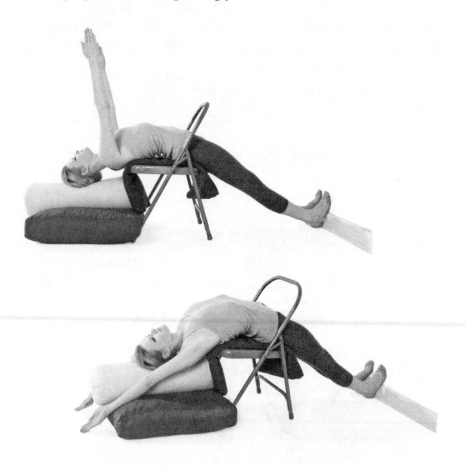

18. To come up, bend your knees and place your feet flat on the floor. Slide back to plant your hips firmly on the chair, and hinge at your hips to sit upright. Keep your chest open and avoid rounding your back.

19. Sit upright for a few breaths to rest before coming out of the chair. Pause to feel the effect of this backbend in your body and mind.

20. To exit the chair, stand up, tip the chair toward the wall, and step out of it.

FULL POSE AT THE WALL

Using the blanket helps to lessen the strain on the wrists yet affords the spine a full extension.

Contraindications: Rotator cuff syndrome, plus all listed in the previous variation.

Avoiding pitfalls: Avoid turning the feet out. Set the arm bones deep into the shoulder sockets to integrate the arms with the spine.

1. Place your mat perpendicular to the wall. Roll the blanket tightly and place it against the wall on your mat.

2. Lie on your back, the top of your head touching the blanket.

3. Place your feet hip-width apart and parallel, knees bent.

4. Place your hands on the blanket roll, shoulder-width apart, with the fingers angled slightly out to the sides.

5. Take a deep breath to broaden your chest and lengthen the sides of the ribs. Engage your arm and leg muscles to prepare to lift yourself up.

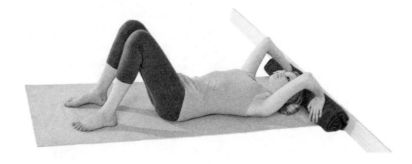

6. Lift your pelvis up, then pick up your shoulders just enough to tuck them under toward your waist, arching your mid-back.

7. Press down again into your feet and hands. Lift your chest enough to put the top of your head on the floor just in front of the blanket roll. Curl your chest toward the wall and your head back.

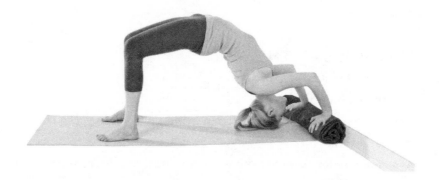

8. Pause to widen your hands if they were not already shoulder-width apart. Adjust your arms deeper into the shoulder joints to make your armpits hollow, and pull your shoulder blades onto your back.

9. Harness all your power, press again through your feet and hands, and push up into a full arch. Your shoulder blades and your tailbone support the lift.

10. Option (not pictured): Lift your heels off the floor to give yourself more space to stretch fully. Be sure to point your knees straight forward.

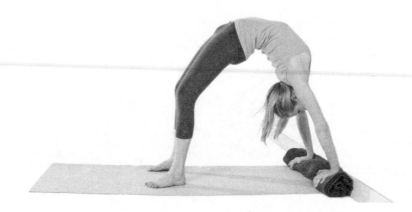

11. Stay in the pose for several quiet breaths, then walk your feet forward and lower yourself down, tucking your chin in toward your chest.

12. Take time to pause and breathe. Absorb the strong stimulus of this backbend.

FULL POSE

Contraindications and pitfalls: See the previous variations.

1. Lie on your back on the mat.

2. Place your feet hip-width apart and parallel, knees bent.

3. Place your hands under your shoulders, with the fingers angled slightly out to the sides.

4. Vigorously pull the arms into the shoulders and the shoulder blades onto the back ribs.

5. Take a deep breath to broaden your chest and lengthen the sides of the ribs.

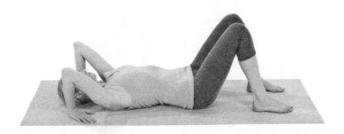

6. Lift your pelvis up, then pick up your shoulders just enough to tuck them under you and toward your waist, arching your mid-back.

7. Press down again into your feet and hands, lifting your chest enough to put the top of your head on the floor. Curl your chest toward your hands and your head back as you do this.

8. Pause to widen your hands if they were not already shoulder-width apart. Adjust your arms deeper into the shoulder joints to make your armpits hollow, and connect your shoulder blades onto your back.

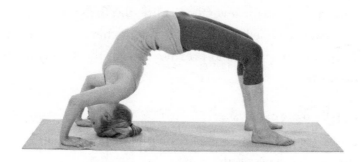

9. Press again through your feet and hands, gathering all your powers to lift up into a full arch. Your shoulder blades and your tailbone help you to lift.

10. Option (not pictured): Raise your heels off the floor to give yourself more space to stretch fully. Be sure to point the knees straight forward.

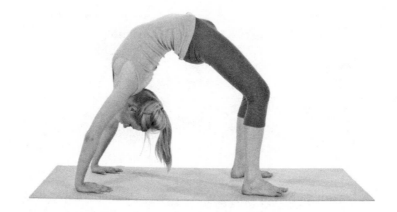

11. Stay in the pose for several breaths, then move your feet forward and lower yourself down, tucking your chin in toward your chest.

12. Take time to pause and breathe, absorbing the strong stimulus of this backbend.

8. JATHARA PARIVARTANASANA
Supine Twist

Purpose: Primarily to apply torque to the anterior lumbar and lateral thoracic and cervical vertebrae, secondarily to generate forces along the lateral thigh bones, anterior lower ribs, and shoulders and to strengthen the abdominal muscles.

Contraindications: Colostomy, inguinal or abdominal hernia, large herniated disc, spondylolisthesis.

Props: A yoga mat, a blanket, a block, and an optional pillow.

Avoiding pitfalls: Maintain maximum length in your spine as you twist. Strongly press your shoulders down onto the floor to stabilize your upper body as the lower body turns.

OSTEOPOROSIS VARIATION

1. Lie on your back on the mat and blanket with your arms outstretched, palms up, and your hips and knees bent 90 degrees. Place the block between your lower legs. Use a pillow to support your head if necessary.

2. Actively widen your sitting bones apart, yet squeeze in on the block with your lower legs. Flex your feet, spreading all ten toes. Lengthen your tailbone and firm your abdomen.

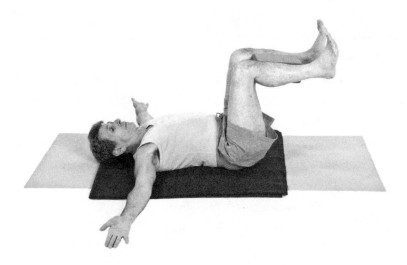

3. Inhale to lengthen your rib cage, then exhale and move your legs to the left, with your shoulders still pressing down.

4. Inhale as you bring your legs back to center.

5. Exhale, move your legs to the right, pressing both shoulders down.

6. Continue to move your legs from left to right several more times,

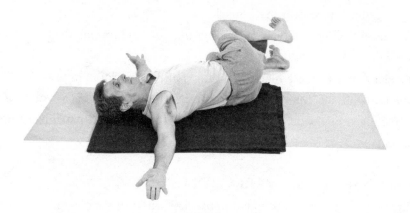

breathing with the actions and pressing your shoulders down into the blanket.

7. Rest on your back with your feet flat, knees bent. Remove the block and breathe deeply.

OSTEOPENIA VARIATION

1. Lie on your back on the mat and blanket with your arms outstretched, palms up, and your knees bent up to your chest. Use a pillow to support your head if necessary.

2. Place a block between your lower legs. Squeeze the block and flex your feet, spreading all ten toes. Lift your feet up so that your knees are open to an angle greater than 90 degrees.

3. Actively widen your sitting bones apart, which will arch your lower back. Then lengthen your tailbone and firm your abdomen.

4. Inhale to lengthen your side ribs, then exhale and move your legs to the left, with your shoulders still pressing down.

5. Inhale as you bring your legs back to center.

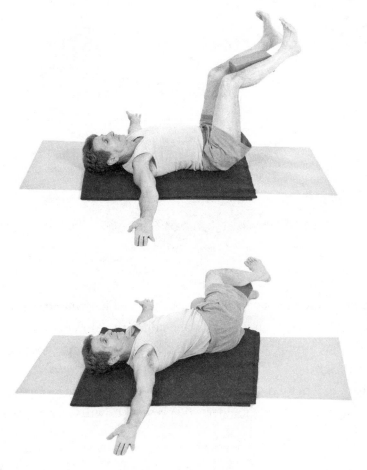

6. Exhale and move your legs to the right, pressing both shoulders down.

7. Continue to move your legs from left to right several more times. Breathe with the actions and press your shoulders down. Relax your neck as much as possible.

8. After several repetitions side to side, rest on your back with your feet flat. Remove the block and breathe deeply to rest.

PREVENTION VARIATION

1. Lie on your back on the mat and blanket with your arms outstretched, palms up.

2. Stretch your legs straight up. Squeeze your legs together and flex your feet. Stretch all your toes.

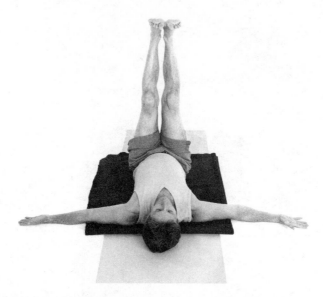

3. Actively widen your sitting bones apart, which will arch your lower back. Then lengthen your tailbone and firm your abdomen.
4. Shift your hips to the left to prepare to counterbalance your legs going to the right.
5. Inhale to lengthen your side ribs, then exhale and move your legs to the right, with your shoulders still pressing down. Go as far as you can

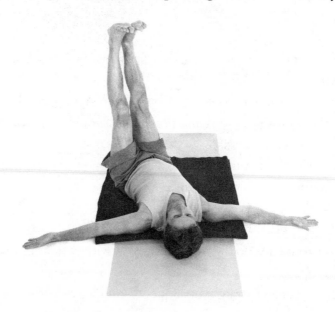

toward the floor without letting the opposite shoulder come up off the floor. Press your right arm down against the floor to lower your left shoulder. Aim your feet toward your right hand. Stay in the pose, ankles together, for 10 to 15 seconds.

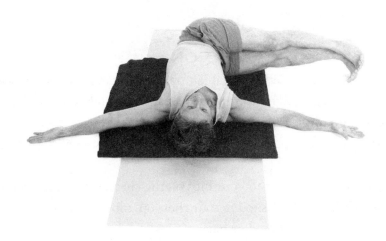

6. Inhale and bring your legs back to center.
7. Exhale and move your legs to the left in the same way, pressing your right shoulder down. Stay in the pose, ankles together, for ten to fifteen seconds.
8. Raise your legs to vertical, then bend your knees and place your feet on the floor in the midline. Breathe deeply to rest. Absorb the stimulus of this strong twist.

9. JANU SIRSASANA
Sitting Forward Stretch

Purpose: To generate isometric anterior-posterior stress on the femurs and all the lumbar and thoracic vertebrae, public rami, and most of the pelvis. Forward bends are quieting, once you get past the initial challenges of tightness. They encourage humility and patience with oneself.

Contraindications: Previous vertebral fracture, colostomy, recently herniated disc.

Props: A yoga mat, a chair, a belt, and a blanket.

Avoiding pitfalls: Press the knee and thigh of the straight leg down and lift your back waist up. Remember to lengthen the spine and avoid rounding.

OSTEOPOROSIS VARIATION

1. Place a chair on your yoga mat. Sit on the front edge of the chair with your right leg straight in front of you and your left knee bent out to the left. Point the right knee straight up.
2. Manually adjust your buttocks and thighs for more width (see pages 87–88).
3. Place your hands next to your hips on the chair seat. Inhale and press down with your hands to lift your chest up, tilting your lower back in and up. Pull your shoulders back.
4. Vigorously stretch your right leg, extending the heel and pulling your toes back toward you.
5. Exhale and incline forward slightly toward your extended leg, leading with your heart. Move forward enough to stretch the back of your right leg well, but take care to avoid curving your spine.

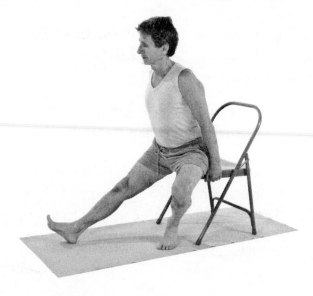

6. Maintain the stretch of your straight leg and the lift of your spine for several breaths, then release.

7. Repeat the pose on the second side.

OSTEOPENIA VARIATION

1. Sit on your mat with your legs outstretched in front of you, a folded blanket under your hips to make the forward tilt of the pelvis easier.

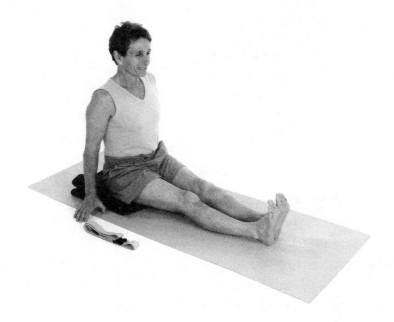

2. Bend your right knee out to the side and place your right foot against the inside of your left upper thigh.

3. Manually reach under your hips and widen the pelvis and upper thighs by pulling the skin and muscles back and out to the side. This will help you tilt your pelvis forward.

4. Tighten the straight leg's quadriceps, pressing the back of the knee and thigh down to the floor and stretching the heel away from you. Stretch your toes up and back toward you to complete the stretch of the leg.

5. Press both sitting bones down and back. Inhale and extend up through the spine.

6. Exhale, hands touching the floor, and turn toward your extended left leg.

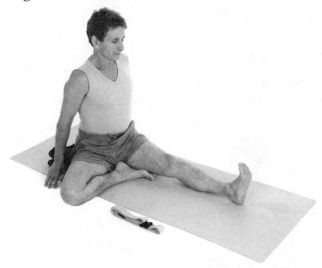

7. Place a belt around your left foot and hold it with your right hand. The left hand on the floor will help you to lift that side of your torso.
8. Inhale and stretch up again.
9. Exhaling, incline forward toward your foot. Keep your arms pulled back into the shoulders even though one is also reaching forward. This will help you to extend the spine without rounding or collapsing it.
10. Shift your belly toward the left to equally lengthen the side ribs, left and right, as you stretch forward toward your foot.

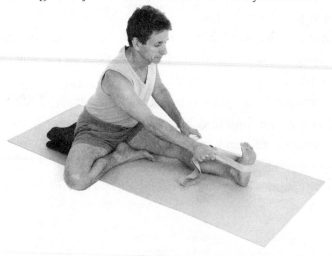

11. Use your breath to remain calm and avoid agitation.

12. Release and repeat on the second side.

PREVENTION VARIATION

1. Follow steps 1–6 above.

7. Place a belt around your left foot and hold it with both hands.

8. Inhale and stretch up again.

9. Exhaling, incline forward toward your foot. Keep your arms pulled back into the shoulders even though they are also reaching forward.

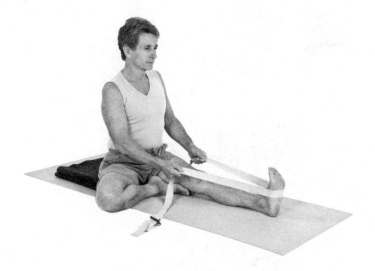

This will help you to extend the spine without rounding or collapsing it.

10. Shift your belly toward the left and equally lengthen the left and right side of the ribs as you stretch forward toward your foot. Pull the right ribs in and turn them toward the left.

11. Use your breath to remain calm and avoid agitation.

12. Don't collapse your back, but keep the front chest lifting as you bend forward. If you are able, grasp your left foot with both hands for a deeper stretch.

13. Release and repeat on the second side.

The following pictures show the full pose. This kind of deep forward bend is not recommended for those with osteoporosis or osteopenia due to the risk of fractures. However, for prevention it is excellent.

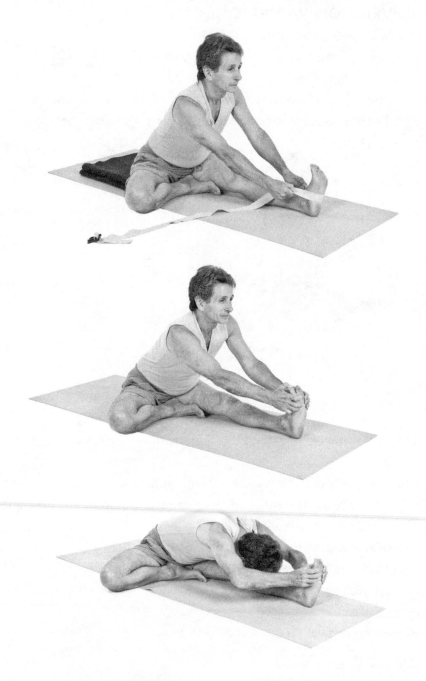

---

10. MARICHYASANA III   Spinal Twist

Purpose: To apply torsion stress to the lumbar and thoracic vertebrae, the shoulder joint, and the femurs from the greater trochanters to the mid-thigh. Twisting poses teach focus and calm even under pressure.

Contraindications: Vulnerability to subluxation/dislocation of the hip or shoulder (for example, after total or partial hip replacement), severe shoulder arthritis, recently herniated disc.

Props: A yoga mat, chair, blanket, and wall.

Avoiding pitfalls: Be mindful of all the alignment details, even if it means that you don't twist as far. Move into the twist with full awareness.

OSTEOPOROSIS VARIATION

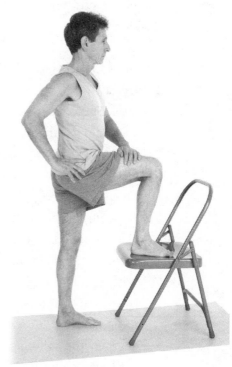

1. Place a chair against a wall. Stand facing the seat of the chair, feet parallel and hip-width apart.
2. Place your right foot on the chair seat, with the knee and foot aligned in front of your hip.
3. Firm your leg and spinal muscles.
4. Widen your sitting bones apart, tilting the top of the pelvis forward slightly.
5. Move the left top thigh back, and resolve to keep it there as you proceed.
6. Lengthen the tailbone down; lift your lower abdomen.
7. Place your right hand on your waist and your left hand on your right thigh.
8. Inhale and stretch up through your spine, and root down through the left leg.
9. Exhale and turn your spine (above the pelvis) to the right. Pull with your left

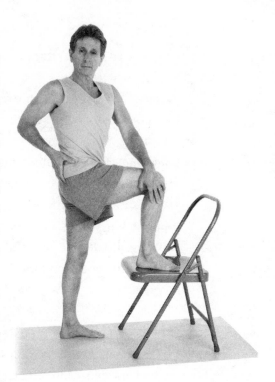

hand on your right knee to help yourself twist. Keep the right thigh firm and wide to resist the pressure of the hand.

10. Actively wrap your left lower ribs around toward the right, beginning with the back ribs, while keeping your left leg firmly rooted. Resist its tendency to move forward. Open your right shoulder back to the right.

11. Keep your shoulders and head level, and work intelligently with moderate effort—not too aggressively, or too gently.

12. Release and repeat on the second side.

OSTEOPENIA VARIATION

1. Place a chair with its right side against a wall. Stand facing its seat, feet parallel and hip-width apart.

2. Place your right foot on the chair seat, with the knee and foot aligned in front of the hip.

3. Firm your leg and spinal muscles.

4. Widen your sitting bones apart, tilting the top of the pelvis forward slightly.

5. Move the left top thigh back, and resolve to keep it there as you proceed.

6. Lengthen the tailbone down and lift your lower abdomen.

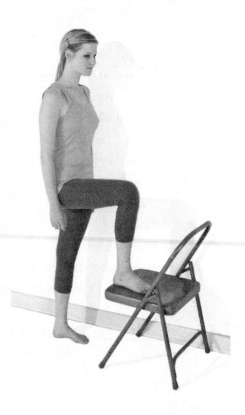

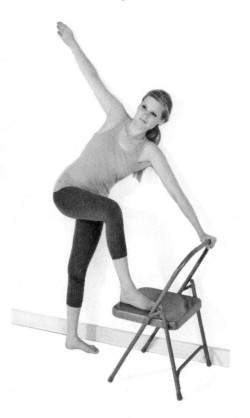

7. Inhale, stretch up through your torso, and exhale as you incline forward by hinging at the hips' joints, spine remaining long. Grasp the chair back with your left hand.

8. Pause to recharge the strength of your legs and spine. Avoid rounding your back.

9. On your next exhalation twist to the right. Pull the right thigh in toward the midline to align it straight forward as you twist.

10. Revolve your right shoulder and spine to the right. Stretch your left hand straight out from your shoulder. Your upper back and shoulders align with the wall.

11. Actively wrap your left ribs around toward the right to originate the twist in the lower torso.

12. Work carefully with moderate effort—not too aggressively, not too gently.

13. Release and repeat on the second side.

PREVENTION VARIATION

1. Sit on the edge of the folded blanket, legs straight forward.

2. Pull your buttocks and upper thighs back and apart to help tip the pelvis forward properly.

3. Breathe to expand inside, strongly lifting the spine up. You can press your hands down on the floor beside you to help the spine lift up.

4. Bend your right knee and place the foot flat on the floor close to the hip.

5. Firmly anchor the left leg down, stretching fully through the sole of the foot. Especially stretch the big-toe side of the foot forward.

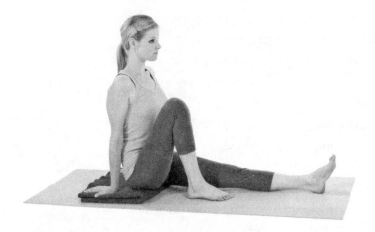

6. On your next inhalation, lift your spine again and turn toward the right. Hook your left elbow on the outside of your right knee. Keep your spine as tall as possible. Point the hand straight up. Your right hand stays on the floor to the side and helps to support your upright spine.

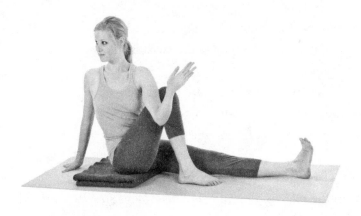

7. Move the spine in and up with your inhalation, and twist more with your exhalation. Lead the twist with your left lower back ribs wrapping toward the right.

8. Within the constriction of the pose, maintain a steady breath and a calm mind.

9. If you feel comfortable, move into the full pose by wrapping the left arm around the bent leg. The right arm wraps around the back, and

you can clasp your hands. This pose requires more flexibility in the spine and shoulders.

10. Release and repeat on the second side.

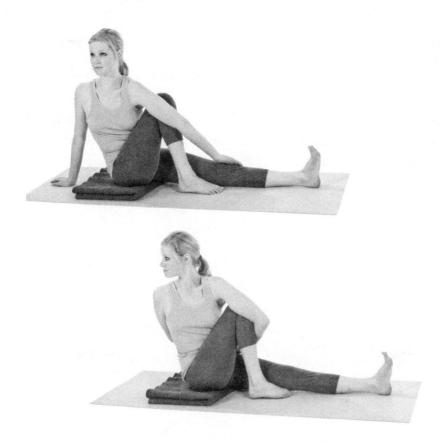

11. PASCHIMOTTANASANA
Hip Fold with Long Spine

Purpose: To stimulate the legs, pelvis, and spine in the anterior-posterior plane, with minimal risk of vertebral fracture in the first variation, and to conclude the practice with a quiet mind. This pose increases patience and steadfastness.

Contraindications: Hamstring sprain, ischial bursitis, recently herniated disc (variations two and three), ischial tunnel syndrome.

Props: A yoga mat, a blanket or two, and one belt.

Avoiding pitfalls: Straighten the legs fully, using a strong contraction of the thigh muscles. In the first variation, press the second leg strongly down onto the floor.

OSTEOPOROSIS VARIATION

This pose is Supta Padangusthasana, an excellent and safe hamstring stretch to prepare for Paschimottanasana.

1. Arrange the folded blanket longitudinally on your mat toward one end. Sit with your buttocks on the mat, at the end of the blanket. Manually spread your buttocks and back thighs apart.

2. Lie down so that the lower edge of the blanket is at the small of your back; the rest of your upper body lies on the blanket. Bend your right knee and place your foot flat on the mat.

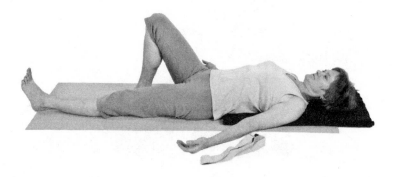

3. Firm the muscles of your legs, pressing the thighs down. Also press the sitting bones down, which will slightly arch your lower back.

4. Contract your abdomen in and up and lengthen your tailbone toward your heels without flattening your lower back.

5. With your pelvis thus stabilized, raise your right leg up and hook a belt around the foot. Hold one end of the belt in each hand.

6. Gradually straighten the leg, firming the muscles on all sides of it, elevating your heel and stretching all five toes. As you do this, continue to press the left leg down onto the floor.

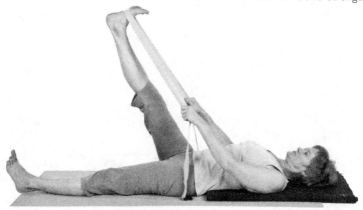

7. Adjust the angle of the right leg so you can straighten your knee. Use your thigh muscles strongly to fully extend the knee.

8. If you cannot straighten the right knee, or if the right leg is not yet at 90 degrees, do the pose with the left leg bent, foot flat on the floor, until your hamstrings become more flexible. This will enable you to stabilize your pelvis.

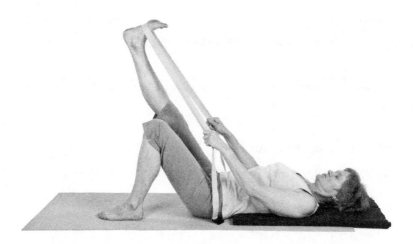

9. If your left leg remains flat on the floor, elongate it by stretching through your heel.

10. For either variation, press the sitting bones down, which will properly tilt the pelvis to achieve the hamstring stretch.

11. The main action is to push your right thigh *away* from your upper

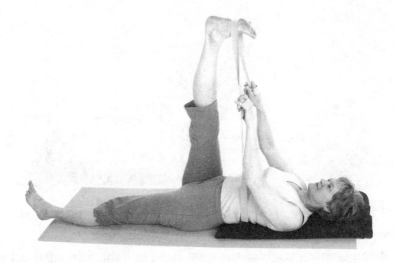

body (which maintains the arch in the lower back), against the resistance of the belt pulling the foot toward you. Note: The goal is *not* to force the right leg or foot toward your head, which will round your lower back.

12. Once you have all the actions going, scan your body for unnecessary tension and release it—especially in the abdomen, shoulders, neck and face.

13. When you are ready, release the right leg down and repeat all steps to stretch the left leg.

OSTEOPENIA VARIATION

1. Sit on the edge of one or two folded blankets with your legs extended forward.

2. Manually pull your sitting bones and thighs back and apart. This will help you to tilt your pelvis forward. Loop the belt around the soles of your feet and hold it with both hands.

3. Hug the leg muscles to the bones and stretch out through your feet, with your toes and kneecaps pointing straight up.

4. Firm your abdominal muscles and lift your spine up from the core of the pelvis, especially the lower back which will tend to round.

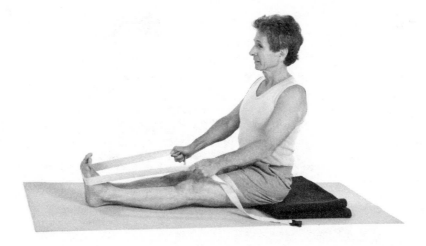

5. Pull on the belt to connect your arms into the shoulders.

6. With each inhalation continue to lift the spine, stretch the legs, and pull your shoulders back.

7. With each exhalation, soften without losing the form or the actions of the pose.

8. Extend up evenly on the sides, front, and back of your torso.

9. Attend to an inner stillness within the dynamic action as you breathe smoothly.

10. When you are ready, release the belt and bend your knees.

PREVENTION VARIATION

1. Follow steps 1–5 above.

6. With each inhalation continue to lift the spine, stretch the legs, and pull your shoulders back.

7. With each exhalation, move forward using a hinging action at your hips not by collapsing your head, shoulders, or chest down. Adjust your hands farther on the belt toward your feet as you are able to progress forward more.

8. Extend up evenly on the sides, front, and back of your torso.

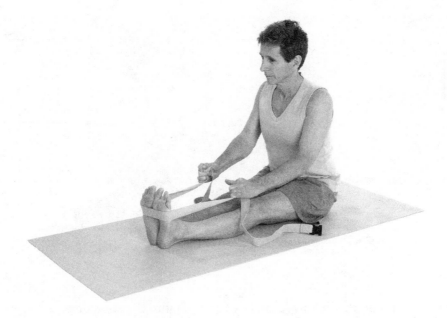

9. Attend to an inner stillness as you breathe smoothly.
10. When you are ready, release the belt, sit upright, and bend your knees.

The full pose is pictured below. It is recommended as preventative stimulus to the vertebrae, but only for those whose flexibility allows them to perform this pose with minimal rounding of the spine.

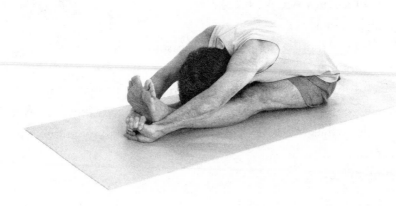

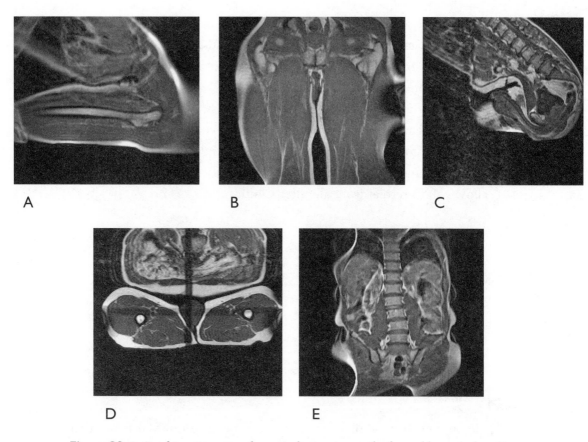

A   B   C

D   E

Figure 32. *In Paschimottanasana the muscular tension on the femoral bones is clear (A, B), the compression of the virtually straight lumbar spine (C) is a preventive antidote to compression fracture, and the alignment of spine and femoral bones tends to equilibrate the forces between them (D). The iliopsoas (E) is completely relaxed in this pose.*

---

12. SAVASANA   Corpse Pose

Purpose: To cease effort, relax, assimilate, and consolidate gains.

Contraindications: Late pregnancy.

Props: A yoga mat, three blankets, optional eye cover.

Avoiding pitfalls: After the initial setup, avoid fussing and fidgeting, become settled. B. K. S. Iyengar commented in *Light on Yoga*, "By remaining motionless for some time and keeping the mind still while you are fully conscious, you learn to relax. This conscious relaxation invigorates and refreshes both body and mind. But it is much harder to keep the mind than the body still. Therefore, this apparently easy posture is one of the most difficult to master."

1. Make sure the space is quiet and safe from distractions.

2. Fold one blanket to support a slight arch of your thoracic spine, roll the second for under your knees, and fold the third one to support your neck and head. An eye cover may help to relax your face and allow you to retreat from all outer stimuli.

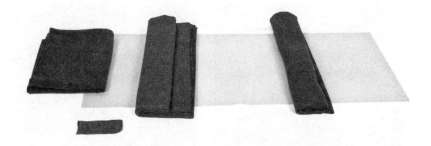

3. Lie on your back with arms at your sides, palms up. Make sure that the chest-supporting blanket allows your shoulders to be flat on the floor. Refold or adjust as necessary.

4. Adjust your hips by turning your legs inward to widen the back of the pelvis, then let the feet roll apart as you relax.

5. Lengthen your buttocks away from the waist if you feel any compression in your lower back.

6. Tuck your shoulder blades gently in toward the spine to open the front of your chest.

7. Make sure that your neck is long and your chin and forehead are level. Then guide your attention through your whole body systematically from head to toe and back again, letting each part relax thoroughly.

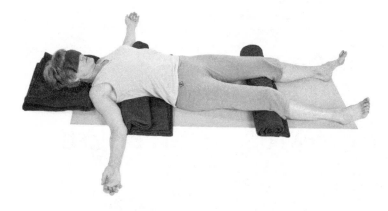

8. Do not fret if your mind produces thoughts; just watch them unemotionally without being drawn into the content. Be a compassionate witness. You might notice yourself reviewing an event, thinking of a person, or making a plan. Try not to follow the pull of any thoughts, but passively observe them come and go. Trust in the process of letting go.

9. After 5 to 10 minutes of quiet rest, take a few deeper breaths, stretch your arms and legs gently, bend your knees, and softly roll to the side. Take your time getting up, and respect whatever effects, changes, and benefits you may feel from your yoga practice. Remember your intention. Affirm your process of growth and healing.

Chapter 10

Poses That Focus on Muscle Strength

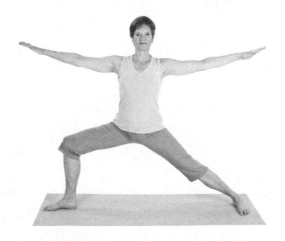

1. VIRABHADRASANA II   Warrior Pose

Purpose: To safely stimulate the femur and pelvic bones using a significant mechanical advantage, improve balance, hip mobility, leg strength, and self assurance.

Contraindications: Anterior cruciate ligament injury, chondromalacia patellae, adductor tear, sacroiliac joint derangement, plantar fasciitis, Achilles tendonitis.

Props: A wall, chair, a block, and a yoga mat.

OSTEOPOROSIS VARIATION

Avoiding pitfalls: If you are tall, use a cushion or block on the chair seat to make it higher. Align the kneecap by pointing it toward the second toe.

1. Place your yoga mat perpendicular to a wall. Place a chair about 18 inches from the wall, facing it.

2. Sit down on the edge of the chair and angle your right knee and foot to the side as much as possible. Your pelvis can turn to the right slightly but attempt to face toward the wall from the waist up.

3. Stretch the left leg off the side of the chair. Turn your left foot and knees slightly in toward the right.

4. Manually adjust your buttocks and thighs back and apart (see pages 87–88).

5. Inhale, lift up from inside, and firm your leg muscles. Straighten the left leg if you can.

6. Exhale. Stay soft in your face and neck but strong in your legs and spine.

7. As you continue to breathe, root down through the pelvic bones, widen your thighs, and lift up through your spine.

8. Rest your hands on the wall and use that directional reference to bring your upper torso to fully face the wall. Pull your shoulders gently back.

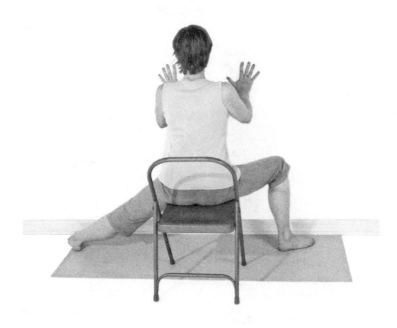

9. It may be some effort to maintain the wide position of the legs, but that effort is what will benefit your pelvic bones.

10. Stay in the pose for as long as you can steadily maintain the actions, then release.

11. Repeat on the second side.

OSTEOPENIA VARIATION

Avoiding pitfalls: Align each foot with its knee, the kneecap pointing toward the second toe. Maintain strong muscular effort in the legs. Bring your feet as wide apart as instructed below; this pose is less effective with a narrow stance.

1. Place your mat along the wall and the chair in front of the middle of the mat, facing away from you. Stand with your back to the wall, raise your arms to shoulder height, and step your feet apart until your ankles are under your outstretched wrists. Once you have established this wide stance, hold the back of chair for balance.

2. Turn your right foot and leg parallel to the wall, but don't turn the torso. Your right hip can lightly touch the wall for reference and support. Line up your right heel with the arch of the left foot.

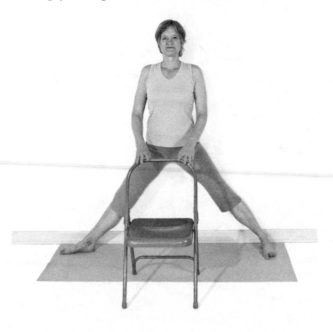

3. Inhale, firm your legs, and lengthen up through the spine. As you exhale, bend your right knee until it is over the ankle. Point the knee toward the second toe.

4. Using the chair for support, lean a bit forward and move both inner groins back.

5. Move the tailbone down and lift your abdomen as you move your torso back up to vertical. This tailbone action initiates an outward rotation of both thighs, but especially the right one. These actions result in the desired effect on your pelvic bones and the safest position for your knees, so be sure to perform them fully.

6. Continue to hold the chair for balance. When you feel steady, spread your arms wide along the wall, palms down. Look to the right, with your head, neck, and spine aligned straight over the center of your pelvis.

7. Hold this position for as long as you can, breathing fully yet smoothly.

8. Repeat on the second side.

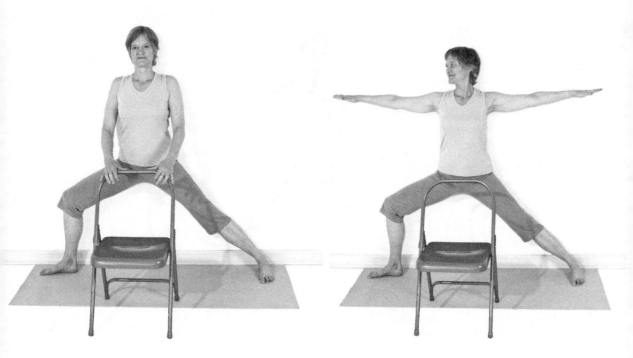

PREVENTION VARIATION USING A WALL

1. Place your mat perpendicular to the wall and the block against the wall.

2. Place your right foot up on the block, toes facing the wall. Step your left foot back until your feet are wide enough apart to be under your wrists when your arms are outstretched. Align the mid-arch of your left foot with your right heel.

3. Inhale, firm your legs, and lengthen up through the spine. As you exhale, bend your right knee until it is over the ankle on the block. Point the knee toward the second toe.

4. Briefly put your hands on your hips. Press down into the very tops of your thighs with your hands to accentuate the bending action there. Lean a bit forward and move both inner groins back.

5. Move the tailbone down and lift your abdomen as you move your

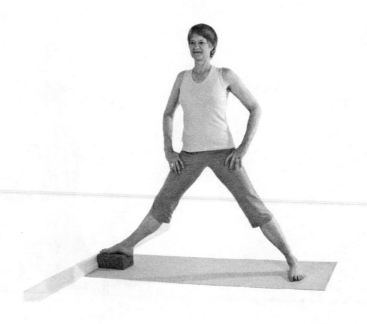

torso back up to vertical. This tailbone action initiates an outward rotation of both thighs, but especially the right one. These actions result in the desired effect on your pelvic bones and the safest position for your knees. Be sure to complete them.

6. Notice that the block under your right foot helps to bring the pelvis level to the floor. This alignment will increase the stretch of both inner thighs considerably.

7. Check to see if the right knee is still facing toward the second toe and that your shin is vertical, knee over the ankle. You may need to step the feet farther apart and turn out the right thigh more to achieve this. In the full pose, the right thigh is parallel to the floor, requiring a very wide stance and deep flexion at the hips and knee. In this variation, the angle at the right knee may be more than 90 degrees.

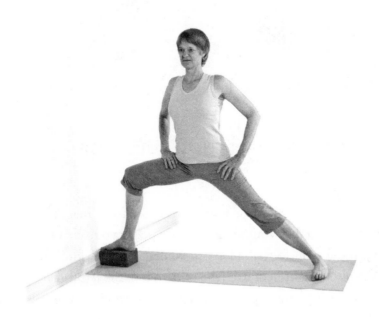

8. Spread your arms wide, palms down, shoulders back. Your right arm may remain bent if it reaches the wall. Look to the right, with your head, neck, and spine aligned straight up over the center of your pelvis. Broaden your upper chest and embody the strength of a warrior, extending out in all directions from the center of your pelvis.

9. Hold for 20 to 30 seconds, breathing fully yet quietly.

10. Repeat on the second side.

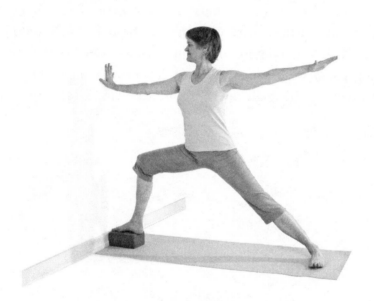

PREVENTION VARIATION FULL POSE

Avoiding pitfalls: Check your alignment in a full-length mirror if possible.

1. Stand on your mat, raise your arms to shoulder height, and step your feet apart so that your ankles line up under your wrists.

2. Turn the right foot and leg out 90 degrees, but don't turn the torso. Align your right heel with the mid-arch of the left foot.

3. Inhale, firm your legs, and lengthen up through the spine. As you

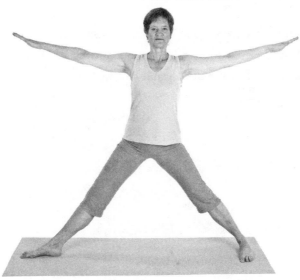

exhale, bend your right knee until it is over the ankle. Point the knee toward the second toe.

4. Check to see that your right knee is turned out sufficiently and that your shin is vertical. You may need to separate the feet farther and turn out the right thigh more to achieve this. In this full version of the pose, the right thigh should be parallel to the floor, requiring a very wide stance and deep flexion at the hips and knee.

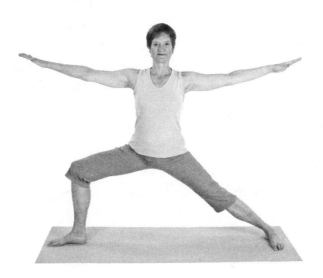

5. Briefly put your hands on your hips. Press down into the tops of your thighs with your hands to accentuate the folding action there. Lean a bit forward and move both inner groins back.

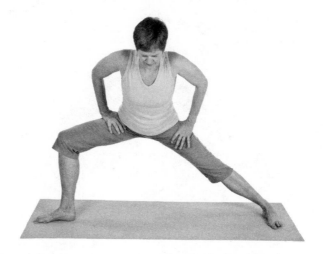

6. Move the tailbone down and lift your abdomen as you move your torso back up to vertical. This tailbone action initiates an outward rotation of both thighs, but especially the right one. These actions increase the forces on your pelvic bones and position the knees safely, so be sure to complete them.

7. Bring your pelvis parallel to the floor; the right side will tend to be lower. This adjustment will increase the stretch of both inner thighs considerably.

8. Spread your arms wide, palms down, shoulders back. Look to the right with your head, neck, and spine aligned straight up over the center of your pelvis. Broaden your upper chest and embody the strength of a warrior, extending out in all directions from the center of your pelvis.

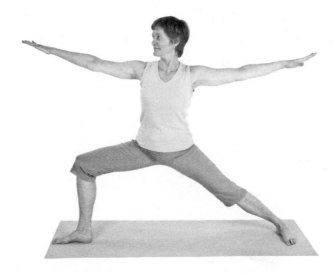

9. Hold for 30 to 60 seconds, breathing fully but softly.

10. Repeat on the second side.

2. PRASARITA PADOTTANASANA
Wide Leg Standing Forward Fold

Purpose: To stretch the adductors, hamstrings, gluteus maximus, and spine; invert the upper body; and stimulate the pelvic and leg bones and vertebral bodies. This wide-open standing pose develops stamina and self-assurance.

Contraindications: Imbalance, ankle sprain, cerebrovascular disease, colostomy, Achilles tendonitis, plantar fasciitis.

Props: A yoga mat and a table.

OSTEOPOROSIS VARIATION

Avoiding pitfalls: Balance your weight on the four corners of your feet and avoid tipping your hips back behind your feet. If you feel strain in your shoulders or arms, place your elbows on the table, shoulder-width apart, instead of your hands. Breathe with ease and fullness, feet facing straight ahead.

1. Place your mat parallel to a table or desk. Stand facing the table and 2 to 3 feet away from it, feet 4 to 5 feet apart, hands on your hips.
2. Inhale, lifting your spine and toning your leg muscles.
3. Exhale, and hinge forward from your hips. Place your hands on the tabletop, shoulder-width apart.

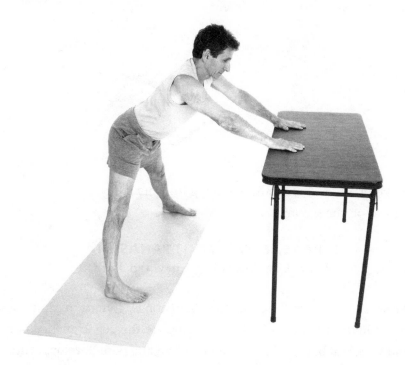

4. On your next exhalation slide your hands forward enough so that your back becomes parallel to the tabletop. Bend your knees to get the proper tilt of your pelvis; there should be one long straight line from your tailbone to the top of your head.
5. Lift your arms and armpits up toward the ceiling as much as possible while keeping your hands firmly on the table.
6. Stretch your sitting bones back and apart. Straighten your knees as much as possible.
7. Firm your abdomen and let your middle back respond to the pull of gravity, softening down without strain.

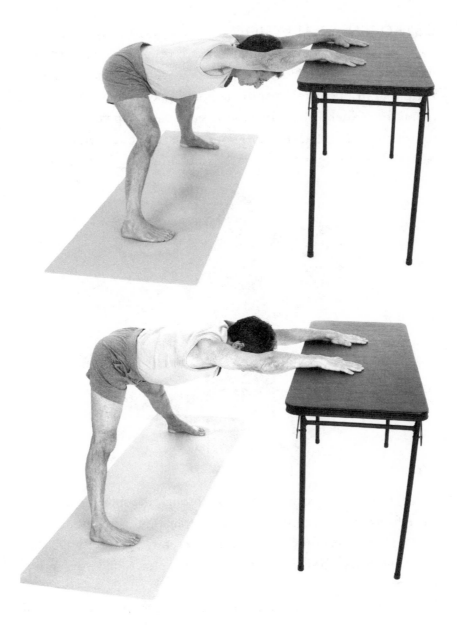

8. Retain the muscular strength in your arms and legs while breathing steadily.

9. When you are ready to come up, walk toward the table. Release your arms down and stand in Tadasana (see page 93).

OSTEOPENIA VARIATION

Avoiding pitfalls: Even when the arms are reaching downward, pull them up into the shoulder sockets. Breathe with ease and fullness.

1. Place your mat perpendicular to the front of a chair. Standing in front of the chair, extend your arms to the sides, then step your feet apart so that your ankles line up under your wrists. Make sure your feet are parallel. Press the four corners of each foot down, but lift your arches.

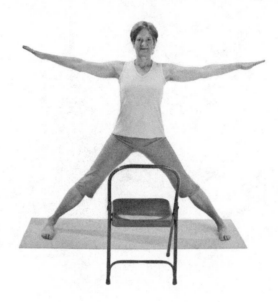

2. Inhale, firm your legs, and stretch up through the spine. Exhale and hinge forward to touch the chair seat, retaining the long spine. You can bend your knees if your hamstrings are very tight. It's important to tip the pelvis forward from your hips; don't round your waist. Reach your hips back.

3. Once your hands are on the chair seat, inhale, extend your legs and sitting bones back, and draw your spine forward. Exhale and release your spine and neck. Repeat this breathing, extending, and releasing movement several times. Then fold your arms and place them on the chair seat. Rest your head on them if possible.

4. As you hold the pose, maintain the strong action in your leg muscles,

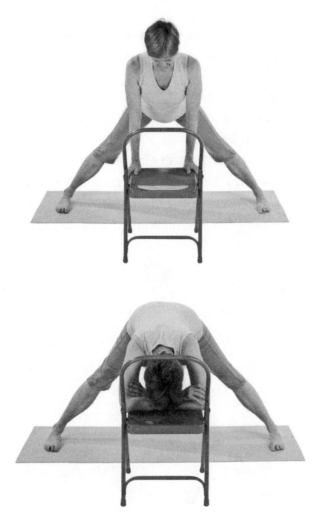

stretching them fully from the feet up to the pelvis. Isometrically widening the thighs laterally will increase the beneficial effect on your bones.

5. Prepare to come out of the pose by stepping your feet a bit closer to each other. Bend your knees and bring your hands to your hips.

6. Inhale and root down through the legs. Stretch your head and chest forward to come up strongly; retract your shoulder blades as you do so.

7. Exhale, step your feet together into Tadasana (see page 93), and release your arms down.

PREVENTION VARIATION

Contraindications: Do not practice this version if you have glaucoma or macular degeneration.

1. Place two blocks about 16 inches in front of the middle of your mat.
2. Extend your arms to the sides, then step your feet apart so that your ankles align under your wrists. Make sure your feet are parallel. Press the four corners of each foot down, but lift your arches.

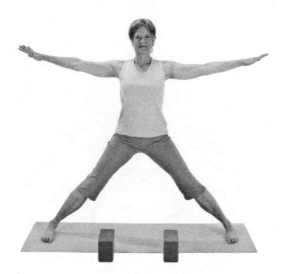

3. Inhale, firm your legs, and stretch up through the spine. Exhale and hinge forward, retaining the long spine, and touch the two blocks. You can bend your knees if your hamstrings are very tight. It's important to tip the pelvis forward from your hips; don't round your waist.
4. Once your hands are on the blocks, inhale, extend your legs and sitting bones back, and draw your spine forward. Exhale and release your spine and neck. Repeat this breathing, extending, and releasing sequence several times. Then bring your spine forward and down,

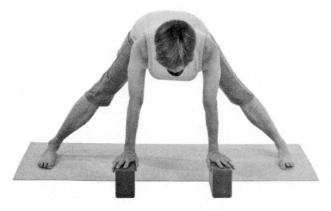

totally releasing your neck and head but keeping your arms pulled up into the shoulder sockets.

5. Maintain the strong lift of your leg muscles. Extend actively from the pelvis out through your legs and up through the crown of your head. Isometrically widening your thighs toward the sides will increase the beneficial effect on your bones.

6. Prepare to come out of the pose by stepping your feet a bit closer to each other. Bend your knees and bring your hands to your hips.

7. Inhale and root down through the legs. Stretch your head and chest forward to come up strongly, retracting your shoulder blades as you do so.

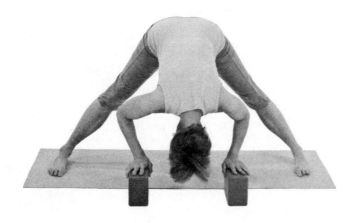

8. Exhale, step your feet together into Tadasana (see page 93), and release your arms down.

The full pose requires more flexibility in the hips. It is pictured for those who are ready for a deeper stretch and who can maintain the length of the spine.

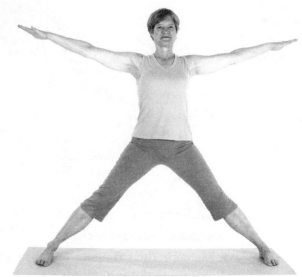

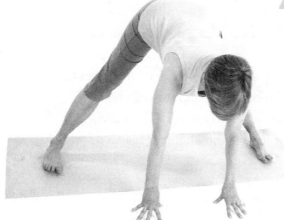

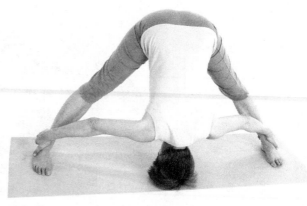

3. PARIGHASANA   Gate Pose

Purpose: Lateral stretch of the torso and leg, stimulating sides of lumbar vertebrae and pelvic bones.

Contraindications: Vertebral fracture, severe lateral listhesis. With moderate or severe scoliosis, only do this pose toward the convex side.

Props: A chair, a blanket, possibly a small rolled towel, a yoga mat, and a wall

Avoiding pitfalls: Be sure to lengthen the spine before bending to the side.

OSTEOPOROSIS VARIATION

1. Place a chair leg-distance from the wall facing to the right.
2. Sit on the left front corner of the chair and extend your left leg toward the wall so that your toes and possibly the entire sole of your foot touch the wall.

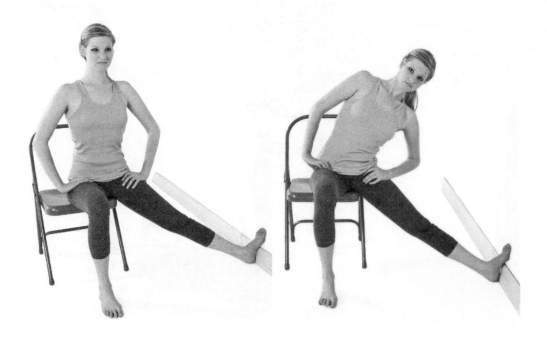

3. Manually widen your buttocks and thighs to ensure that your pelvis will sit upright on the chair, not slumped backward.

4. Inhale and stretch up through your spine. Firm the leg muscles, keeping the left leg straight.

5. Firm and lift your abdominal muscles up. Lengthen the tailbone down.

6. Place your hands on the tops of your thighs.

7. As you exhale, incline your torso to the left, maintaining length through the crown of your head. As you lean more to the left, slide your hand down your left leg.

8. Widen your front chest and pull your shoulder blades together as you extend through the entire spine.

9. Hold for several breaths, then return to vertical as you inhale.

10. Repeat on the second side.

OSTEOPENIA VARIATION

1. Spread a blanket on your mat and place a chair on the left end of the mat facing in.

2. Kneel on the blanket with your legs slightly apart, feet stretching straight back. If your feet are stiff, place a small rolled towel under your right ankle (not pictured).

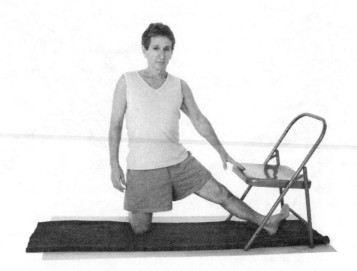

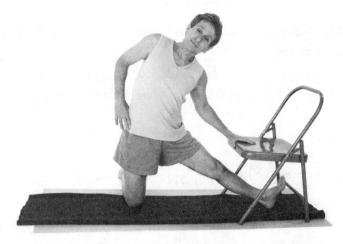

3. Extend your left leg out to the side, under the chair against the back rung.
4. Inhale and straighten the left leg. Stretch all the way through your toes.
5. Stretch up through the sides of your body to prepare to bend to the side.
6. On your next exhalation, bend your torso to the left. Place your left hand or forearm on the chair seat for support. Your right hand rests on your hip. Take several breaths.
7. When you are ready, swing your right arm out to the side, up and over toward the left, reach well beyond the right side of your head.

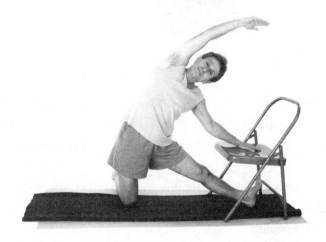

8. Remain solidly grounded through your pelvis and legs as you reach more and more.

9. Hold for several breaths, then inhale to come up. Notice the increased space in your rib cage from this stretch, which will improve your breathing.

10. Repeat on the second side.

PREVENTION VARIATION

1. Place your yoga mat perpendicular to a wall, and spread a blanket on the mat. Kneel on the blanket with your legs slightly apart and your shins and feet parallel to the wall on your left.

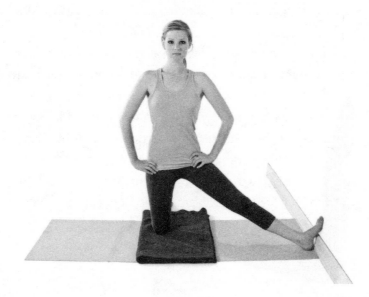

2. Stretch your left leg out to the side without turning your pelvis; less than 90 degrees to the side is fine. Put the ball of your foot on the wall.

3. Inhale, stretch your left leg straight, and lengthen up through your torso.

4. Raise your arms to shoulder height and turn the right palm up.

5. Firm and lift your abdominal muscles, root the tailbone down, and lean slightly forward.

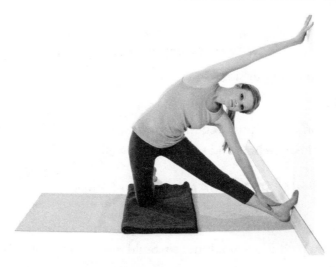

6. On your next exhalation, bend to the left. Slide your left hand down your leg. Raise your right arm up and over toward your extended leg, touching the wall if possible.

7. Avoid collapse in the upper back by pulling your shoulder blades in toward the spine. Face forward as much as possible.

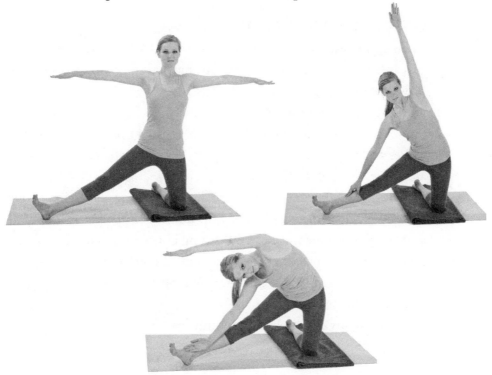

8. After several breaths in the pose, use an extra measure of strength to come back up to vertical. Notice how your breathing feels after this strong stretch of your ribs.

9. Repeat on the second side.

The full version of this pose requires more strength and flexibility, and will stimulate the vertebrae and pelvic bones well.

4. USTRASANA   Camel Pose

Purpose: To stimulate the anterior and posterior vertebrae, anterior pelvis, femur and acetabulum; to build upper body strength and confidence.

Contraindications: (absolute) severe spondylolisthesis or spondylitis; (relative) severe ventral hernia, severe spinal stenosis, anterior cruciate ligament tear, patellofemoral arthralgia, chondromalacia patella.

Props: A yoga mat, a blanket, a bolster, and a chair.

OSTEOPOROSIS VARIATION

Avoiding pitfalls: Make sure the shoulders are back and your spine and ribs are elongated before you lift your hips off the chair. If your arms or wrists are weak, practice only steps 1–3.

1. Place a chair on your mat.

2. Sit on the front edge of the chair. Step your feet out about eighteen inches and place them hip-width apart. Place your hands on the seat, alongside or slightly behind your hips.

3. Inhale and lift up from inside, gradually lengthening and arching your spine. Breathe to the very top of your lungs. Your pelvis tips forward at the top near your waist as your sitting bones move back and apart.

4. Pull your shoulders back; the shoulder blades move toward the spine.

5. On your next inhalation, lift your hips off the chair, moving your knees and thighs forward.

6. Look up slightly and breathe smoothly.

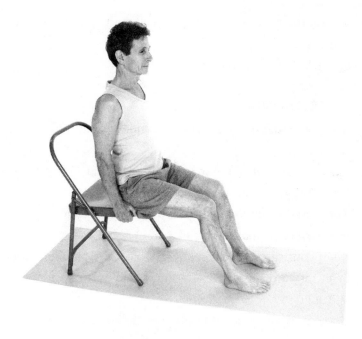

7. As you push down through your arms, lift your chest more. The downward thrust of your arms and the upward thrust of your hips and chest balance each other.

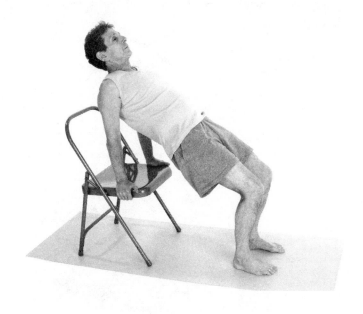

8. Stay in the pose for as long as you can maintain the lift of your hips and chest.

9. Sit back down on an exhalation and rest.

OSTEOPENIA VARIATION

Avoiding pitfalls: Press your foundation down to lift your spine strongly.

1. Place a chair on one end of your mat, seat facing in. Place a folded blanket on the mat, extending under the chair.

2. Kneel on the blanket with your back to the chair, legs hip-width apart, feet under the chair seat.

3. Align your calves and feet straight back and parallel. Spread your toes.

4. Lean forward slightly and isometrically push your upper thighs back and apart.

5. Come upright again and pull your tailbone down.

6. Lift up through the mid-torso and ribs to prevent compression of the lumbar vertebrae as you bend backward. Place your hands on your hips and press the pelvis down as you lift the spine up. This will accentuate the dynamic action.

7. Retract your shoulder blades toward the spine and begin reaching behind you.

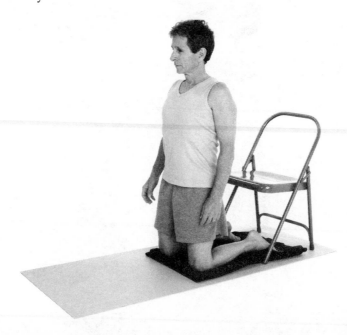

8. Inhale and vigorously lift your heart and lungs.

9. Grasp the chair seat or legs. Slowly and sequentially arch your middle back, upper back, and chest.

10. Arch your head and neck, first from the base of your head, then your ears, then the top of your head.

11. These actions will support and guide you: press your lower legs into the floor and your tailbone forward, lift your heart up, and continue to breathe fully and smoothly.

12. To exit the pose, lift your head and shoulders upright, then walk your legs out from under the chair and sit down on your heels.

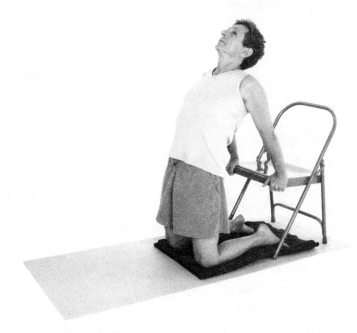

PREVENTION VARIATION

Avoiding pitfalls: Tilt only minimally to one side as you reach back.

1. Place a folded blanket on your mat. Kneel on the blanket, legs hip-width apart, and place a bolster over your ankles.

2. Align your calves and feet straight back and parallel. Spread your toes.

3. Lean forward slightly and isometrically push your upper thighs back and apart.

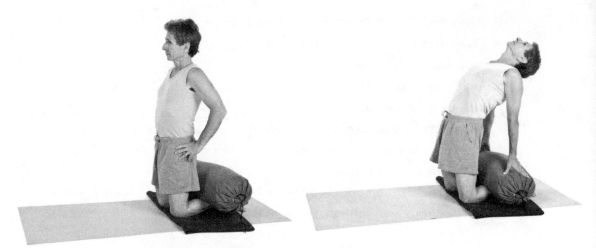

4. Come upright again and pull your tailbone down.

5. Lift up through the mid-torso and ribs to prevent compression of the lumbar vertebrae as you bend backward. Place your hands on your hips and press the pelvis down as you lift the spine up. This will accentuate the two-directional action.

6. Retract your shoulder blades toward your spine and begin to reach your arms behind you.

7. Inhale and vigorously lift your heart and lungs.

8. Reach for the bolster with your hands. Slowly and sequentially arch your middle back, upper back, and chest.

9. Arch your head and neck, first from the base of your head, then your ears, then the top of your head.

10. Continue these supportive actions as you stay in the pose: Press your lower legs into the floor and your tailbone forward, lift your heart up, and continue to breathe fully and smoothly from the lower chest to the upper chest.

11. To exit the pose, lift your head and shoulders upright, then sit down on your heels.

For the full version of this pose, your hands come onto your feet. All the actions described above apply here as well.

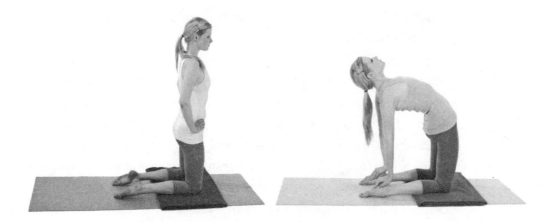

5. ADHO MUKHA SVANASANA
Downward Facing Dog

Purpose: To stress the posterior thigh and shin bones, calcaneus, inner humerus, forearm bones, wrists, shoulder blades, lower anterior ribs, and posterior elements of all vertebrae. This is a particularly invigorating pose.

Contraindications: Acromioclavicular dysfunction, rotator cuff tear, thoracic outlet syndrome, spondylolisthesis, Dupuytren's contractures, carpal tunnel syndrome, Achilles tendon tear.

Props: A yoga mat, wall, and chair.

Avoiding pitfalls: Retract the shoulder blades firmly onto the back ribs; don't let the upper arms sag downward. Roll the inner arms upward toward the ceiling to maintain the proper rotation of the upper arms. This will help to firm your elbows in toward the midline, providing stability in the pose. Keep the knees bent if you are stiff, in order to be able to tilt the pelvis and lengthen the spine.

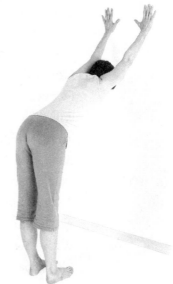

OSTEOPOROSIS VARIATION

1. Place your yoga mat next to a wall. Stand 12 to 14 inches from the wall and place your hands on the

wall above eye level, index fingers pointing up and the arms shoulder-width apart.

2. Place your feet hip-width apart and parallel.

3. Straighten your arms and move your chest a little toward the wall.

4. Move your upper arms more securely back into the shoulder joints.

5. Keep your elbows straight and your upper arms light but active.

6. Bend forward through your trunk until there is one long diagonal line from hands to hips. You can step back as needed. Do not round your back.

7. Stretch back with your sitting bones and separate them, which will make an arch in your lower back.

8. Draw in your belly and lengthen the tailbone back.

9. Let the thoracic spine soften downward without collapsing your arms.

10. If your hamstrings allow, do the pose with straight legs. If your hamstrings are tight, your knees can be bent slightly in order to allow the pelvis to tilt properly. Find the degree of effort in extending yourself that feels good, using your breath.

11. After several breaths, come back up as you inhale and step toward the wall.

OSTEOPENIA VARIATION

1. Place a chair against the wall, facing out toward you. Place your mat in front of the chair.

2. Hold the front outer edges of the chair seat and walk your feet back, feet remaining hip-width apart and parallel. How far you step back will vary according to your flexibility; go as far as you can without losing stability.

3. Bend your knees as you reach your hips back to stretch the spine and arms in one long line from hands to hips.

4. Breathe fully into the sides of the rib cage and maintain strength in all parts of the body. Your head stays between your arms.

5. With each inhalation, reach your sitting bones up, back and apart. Make space.

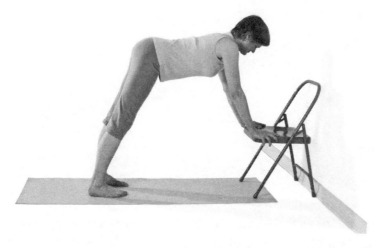

6. With each exhalation, elongate all the lines of the pose (legs, arms, spine). Expand out strongly from the inside.

7. Stretch your legs straight, if you can do so without curling the back of the pelvis down. You can step back farther, and your heels can be off the floor.

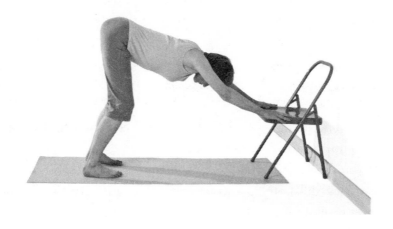

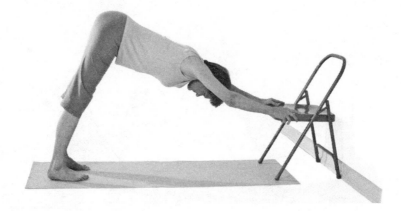

8. Hold the pose for several breaths. To come out of the pose, walk toward the chair and stand up.

PREVENTION VARIATION

1. Come down onto your hands and knees on your mat. Walk your knees back a bit farther than your hips. Place your hands at the front of the mat, shoulder-width apart, fingers separated, index fingers pointing forward.

2. Firm your arm muscles, press your fingers down, and soften your chest down over the tops of the arms so that the arms connect solidly into the shoulder sockets.

3. Draw your shoulder blades in toward your spine.

4. Tuck your toes under and make space in the sides and front of your entire torso.

5. Inhale and lift up your knees and hips, elevating the sitting bones back, up and apart.

6. As you exhale, stretch fully through your arms and spine, pulling your legs back still farther. If your hamstrings are very tight, bend your knees to allow your pelvis to tilt properly. Gradually work to straighten your knees.

7. Create a slight concavity in the lumbar and thoracic spine by reaching upward with the sitting bones.

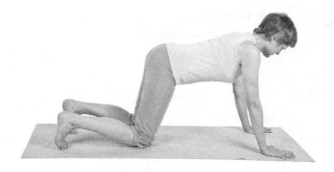

8. As you become more flexible, you will be able to pull the thighs back with straight knees, and eventually lower your heels.

9. Once you have created the full pose, sensitively extend through all parts of the body, from the core to the periphery. Charge your body with strength.

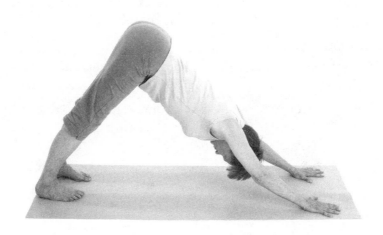

10. To release, bring your knees to the floor.

6. CHATURANGA DANDASANA
Four-Limbed Staff Pose

Purpose: To strengthen the upper back and arms; to stimulate the cervical, thoracic, and lumbar vertebrae, as well as ankles, hips, shoulders, and wrists; to build core strength.

Contraindications: Carpal tunnel syndrome, severe wrist arthritis, Dupuytren's contracture.

Props: A wall, a chair, a yoga mat, and a blanket.

Avoiding pitfalls: Make sure to retract your shoulder blades and broaden your front chest. Shoulders should stay square across and the whole body remain in one long line. Check using a mirror or a friend. Use your abdominal muscles to maintain the alignment of the body's midsection.

OSTEOPOROSIS VARIATION

1. Stand facing a wall, about 18 inches from it, with your hand at about mid-chest height on the wall and shoulder-width apart. Point your index fingers straight up.
2. Draw your upper arms back and firm your shoulder blades onto the back ribs.
3. Lengthen your tailbone down. Connect the whole length of your

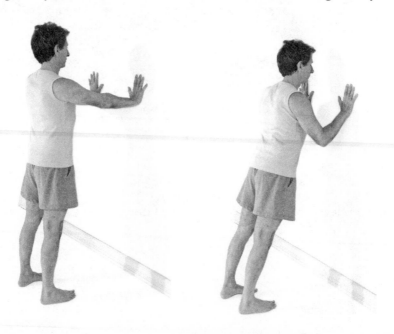

body into one long energetic line that expands out from the pelvis, stretching downward through your feet and upward through the crown of your head.

4. Inhale to prepare.

5. Exhale and bend your elbows, inclining the whole length of your body toward the wall.

6. Check yourself: Are your shoulders staying back or did they round forward? Keep them back. Did your pelvis move toward the wall with you? Don't allow it to hang back.

7. Move in and out several times, then hold the pose for as long as you can while you are inclined toward the wall.

8. Return to vertical and release your hands down.

OSTEOPENIA VARIATION

1. Place your yoga mat perpendicular to a wall. Place a chair with its back to the wall and a folded blanket on the floor in front of it.

2. Kneel on the blanket and place your hands on the sides of the chair.

3. Firm your abdominal muscles and pull your tailbone down. The pelvis easily becomes misaligned in this pose, and it is important to support it with firm muscular control.

4. Inhale, pull your shoulders back, and lengthen from your knees to the top of your head.

5. Exhale, bend your elbows, and incline yourself toward the chair seat, maintaining a straight line from your knees to the top of your head.

6. Check yourself: Are your shoulders staying back or did they round forward? Keep them back. Did your pelvis move toward the chair

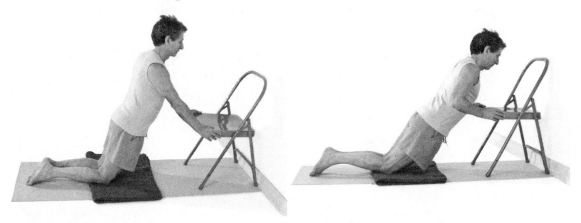

with you? Don't let it hang back. Align your upper arms with the sides of your torso.

7. Move in and out several times, then hold the pose for as long as you can while you are inclined toward the chair, up to a full minute. Continue to breathe evenly and quietly.

8. Return to vertical and release your hands down.

PREVENTION VARIATION

1. Kneel with your hands shoulder-width apart on the mat under your shoulders. Your index fingers point forward.

2. Move your hands forward one hand's length.

3. Tip your tailbone slightly down and firm your abdominal muscles. Move the sides of your waistline back. This supports the alignment of the body's midsection, which tends to collapse.

4. Inhale, retract your shoulders, and lengthen from your hips to the top of your head.

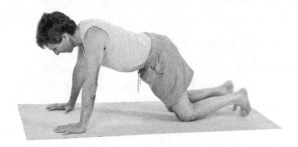

5. Exhale, bend your elbows, and incline yourself toward the floor, maintaining a straight line from your knees to the top of your head. Keep your shoulders back.

6. If possible, lower down enough to bring your upper arms alongside your ribs. Gaze toward the floor, and keep your neck long.

7. Check yourself: Are your shoulders staying back or did they round forward? Keep them back. Did your pelvis move forward with you? Don't let it hang back.

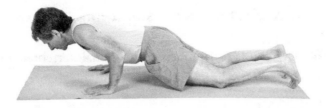

9. Pause for a few seconds in the pose, then release to the floor and rest. Congratulate yourself: This is a very challenging pose!

The full version of this pose, requiring more strength, begins from the same hands-and-knees position, then moves to Plank Pose. Finally the entire body is lowered until it hovers above the floor, with the shoulders remaining back and the abdomen strong. The most common misalignment is for the pelvis to be too high and the head and shoulders too low, so have a friend check your position.

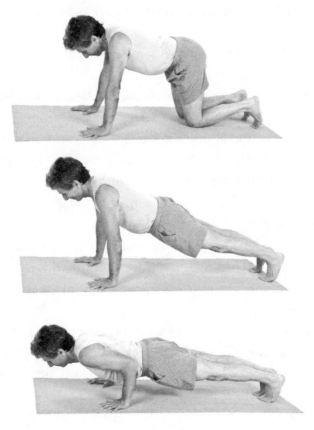

7. ANANTASANA   Side-Lying Balance

Purpose: To stimulate the sides of the spinal vertebrae and the iliac and femoral bones; to improve balance; and to enhance lower extremity circulation.

Contraindications: Trochanteric bursitis, tardy ulnar palsy, facet syndrome, medial epicondylitis.

Props: A wall, a yoga mat, a belt, and an optional blanket.

Avoiding pitfalls: Draw your muscles into the core of your body; when the body is integrated by this muscular action, it's easier to find the balance. Keep as much contact with the wall as needed.

OSTEOPOROSIS VARIATION

1. Place your mat alongside a wall and spread a blanket on it if you want more padding. Lie on the floor on your right side with your back to the wall.

2. Stack your left leg on top of your right with the feet touching each other on the big-toe side.

3. Extend your right upper arm parallel to the wall, bend the elbow, and rest your head in your hand, looking out away from the wall. Your left shoulder can lean against the wall for support.

4. Place your left hand in front of you on the floor for balance.

5. Inhale and firm the muscles in your legs and torso. Continue to breathe normally. Maintain this muscular support for the entire duration of the pose.

6. Lift your left leg up away from the right leg just a few inches and hold it there. Press your right leg down into the floor. This action pulls directly on the greater trochanter, the part of the hip that commonly fractures.

7. In addition to holding your leg up and balancing your torso on its side, extend actively through both legs with a strong stretch from your pelvis all the way out through your toes. Extend the spine from the pelvis out through the crown of your head.

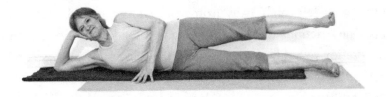

8. Hold the pose for as long as you can, then rest.
9. Repeat on the second side.

OSTEOPENIA VARIATION

1. Place your mat alongside a wall and spread a blanket on it if you want more padding. Lie on the floor on your right side with your back to the wall.
2. Bend your legs, bringing your knees slightly away from the wall, feet against the wall.
3. Extend your right upper arm parallel to the wall, bend the elbow, and rest your head in your hand, looking out away from the wall. Your left shoulder can rest on the wall for support.
4. Loop a belt around your left foot.
5. Turn your left knee up toward the ceiling and stretch the foot up, holding the belt with your left hand. Straighten the knee if possible.
6. Inhale and firm all the muscles in your legs and torso. Press the right leg into the floor to counterbalance the left leg going up. Continue to breathe normally. Maintain this muscular support for the duration of the pose.

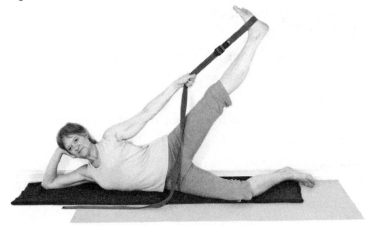

7. Press your left thigh away from your shoulders and stretch the heel up. These actions will help to straighten the knee more and more.

8. In addition to holding your leg up and balancing your torso on its side, extend actively through your left leg with a strong stretch from your pelvis all the way out through your toes. Extend the spine from the pelvis out through the crown of your head. This expansion will help you balance.

9. Hold for as long as you can, up to one minute, breathing and remaining steady, then bring the left leg down and rest.

10. Repeat on the second side.

PREVENTION VARIATION

1. Place your mat alongside the wall and spread a blanket on it if you want more padding. Lie on the floor on your right side with your back to the wall.

2. Stack your left leg on top of your right with the feet touching each other on the big-toe side.

3. Extend your right upper arm parallel to the wall, bend the elbow, and rest your head in your hand, looking out away from the wall.

4. Place your left hand in front of you on the floor for balance.

5. Inhale and firm the muscles in your legs and torso. Continue to breathe normally. Maintain this muscular support for the entire duration of the pose.

6. Lift your left leg up away from the right leg, bend the knee, and turn it toward the ceiling. Press the right leg against the floor to counterbalance the left leg going up.

7. Hook the belt around your left foot and straighten the knee as much as possible. Turn your leg so that the knee and toes face straight toward your head.

8. Press your left thigh away from your shoulders and stretch the heel up. These actions will help to straighten the knee.

9. In addition to holding your leg up and balancing your torso on its side, extend actively through both legs with a strong stretch from your pel-

vis all the way out through your toes. Extend the spine from the pelvis out through the crown of your head. These actions pull directly on the greater trochanter, the part of the hip that commonly fractures.

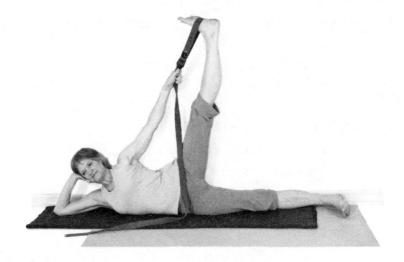

10. Play with balancing without the support of the wall.
11. Hold for as long as you can, then rest.
12. Repeat on the second side.

The full pose is more challenging when practiced without a belt away from the wall. All the same preparatory steps apply.

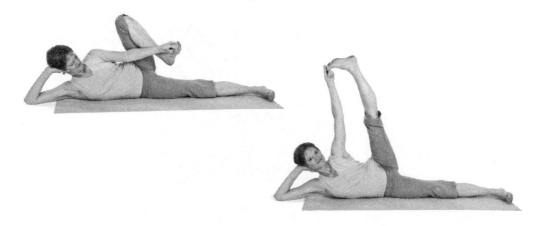

8. PARIPURNA NAVASANA Boat Pose

Purpose: To stimulate the anterior lumbar vertebrae, pelvic bones, and femur; to improve strength, balance, and focus.

Contraindications: Herniated disc, piriformis syndrome, ischial bursitis, hamstring tear.

Props: A yoga mat, a chair, and a blanket.

Avoiding pitfalls: Keep your chest fully lifted; don't round forward.

OSTEOPOROSIS VARIATION

1. Place your mat perpendicular to a wall. Place a chair back against the wall, and a blanket on the mat in front of it.
2. Sit on the blanket, your back a few inches away from the edge of the chair, your knees bent, and your feet flat.
3. Hold your legs behind the knees.
4. Inhale, pull your shoulders back, and lift up your spine and chest.
5. Tip your pelvis so the waistline comes forward toward your legs. All your lumbar and thoracic paraspinal muscles will be working.
6. Firm your abdominal muscles to support your spine from the front.
7. Exhale and lean back, touching the chair lightly with your upper back, and bring your feet off the floor. You will be balanced on your sitting

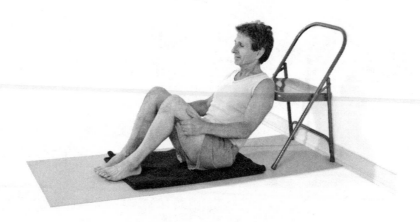

bones. Take care not to slump forward. You can try it first with just one foot lifting, then add the second foot when ready.

8. Lengthen your spine from the pelvis to the crown of your head and stretch your feet, spreading the toes.

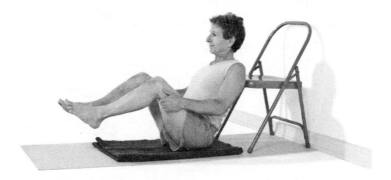

9. Continue to breathe smoothly and fully as you hold the pose for about 30 seconds, then release and sit comfortably to rest.

OSTEOPENIA VARIATION

1. Sit on your mat with your knees bent, heels on the floor. Place your hands behind you on the floor and lift up your spine.
2. Keep your spine lifted as you place your hands behind your knees.
3. Inhale, pull your shoulders back, and lift up your spine and chest.
4. Tip your pelvis to arch your lower back and bring your waistline

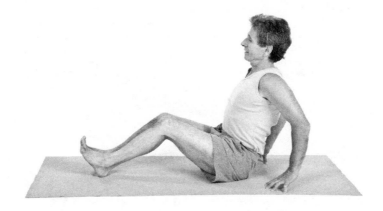

forward toward your legs. All your lumbar and thoracic paraspinal muscles will be working.

5. Firm your abdominal muscles to support your spine and keep it long.

6. Exhale and lean back, bringing your feet off the floor. You will be balanced on your sitting bones.

7. Raise your lower legs until they are parallel to the floor. Flex your feet and stretch through all ten toes.

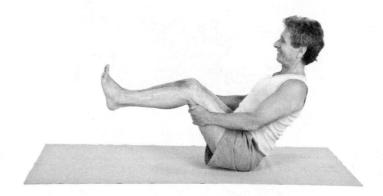

8. Lengthen your spine from the pelvis to the crown of your head.

9. If you feel steady enough, release your hands from your knees and stretch your arms horizontally. Only do this when you can keep your spine extended.

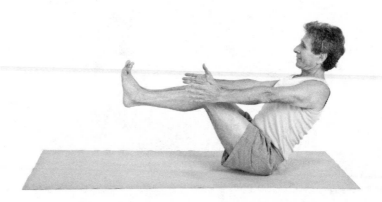

10. Continue to breathe smoothly and fully as you hold the pose for about 30 seconds, then release and sit comfortably to rest.

PREVENTION VARIATION

1. Sit on your mat. Manually adjust your buttocks back and apart (see pages 87–88).
2. Bend your knees up and heels on the floor, place your toes extending upward. Place your hands behind you on the floor.
3. Inhale, pull your shoulders back, and lift up your spine and chest.
4. Tip your pelvis to arch your lower back and move your waistline forward toward your legs. All your lumbar and thoracic paraspinal muscles will be working.

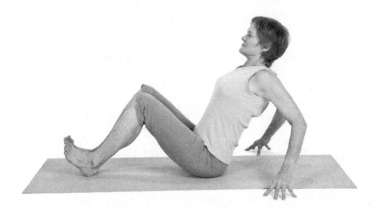

5. Firm your abdominal muscles to support your spine from the front.
6. Inhale and lean back, bringing your feet off the floor. You will be balanced on your sitting bones. Hold the backs of your legs.
7. Stretch your legs out to a 45-degree angle so that you are looking at the middle of your shins. Flex your feet and stretch through all ten toes.
8. Extend your arms alongside your legs, parallel to the floor. Pull the shoulders back even as you reach the hands forward.
9. Lengthen your spine from the pelvis to the crown of your head and continue to fully stretch your arms and legs.

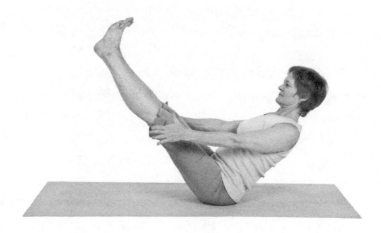

10. Breathe smoothly and fully as you hold the pose for about 30 seconds, then release and sit comfortably to rest.

9. ARDHA MATSYENDRASANA
Classic Seated Twist

Purpose: This pose puts a resistive load on the entire skeleton, one side at a time.

Contraindications: Herniated lumbar disc, spondylolisthesis, vertebral fracture, colostomy, rotator cuff tear.

Props: A yoga mat, a chair, a wall, and a blanket.

Avoiding pitfalls: Lengthen the spine upward to free it and the rib cage for rotation. Root down through the pelvic bones. Use your abdominal muscles to help you twist.

OSTEOPOROSIS VARIATION

1. Place a chair with its left side about 6 inches from a wall. Sit down and cross your left leg over your right.
2. Manually widen your buttocks and thighs (see pages 87–88). This will help avoid a slumped posture. Your sitting bones move back and apart.
3. As you inhale, lift your spine up and root down through the pelvic bones. Isometrically widen your thighs apart even though they

will not move. This action will provide a base from which the spine will twist fully. It also pulls strongly on the pelvic bones.

4. As you exhale, firm your abdominal muscles, lengthen your tailbone down, and turn toward the wall. Place your right hand on your left knee and your left hand on the wall wherever it is comfortable. Push your left hand into the wall for the leverage to twist to the left. Bring the right chest forward more than the shoulder.

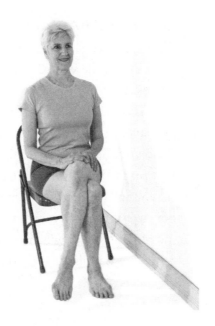

5. Using your arms and legs strongly, carefully create the power for a deep twist of the spine. Retain a vertically elongated spine; do not tilt your head.

6. Continue to breathe and soften internally to receive the twist. There may be a subtle inner turn still possible even when your spine and ribs seem to have reached their limit.

7. After several breaths, return to face your knees and uncross your legs.

8. Repeat on the second side.

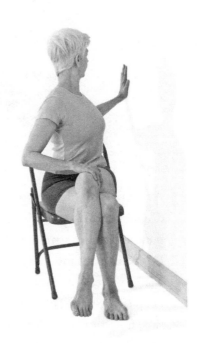

9. After completing both sides, sit for a moment to feel the effects of this pose, which does its work in so many areas of the body.

OSTEOPENIA VARIATION

1. Place your yoga mat alongside a wall, and a blanket on it about 6 inches from the wall. Sit on the blanket with your left side to the wall and extend your legs forward.
2. Manually widen your buttocks and thighs (see pages 87–88). This will help avoid a slumped posture. Your sitting bones move back and apart.
3. Bend your left knee, cross the left leg over the right, and place the left foot on the floor to the outside of your right leg.
4. As you inhale, lift your spine up and root down through your pelvic bones. Isometrically widen your thighs even though they will not move. This action will provide a base from which your spine will twist fully. It also pulls strongly on the pelvic bones.

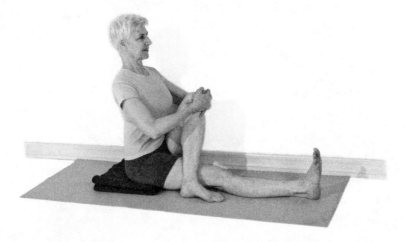

5. As you exhale, firm your abdominal muscles, lengthen your tailbone down, and turn toward the wall. Grasp your left knee with your right hand or folded arm and place your left hand on the wall behind you. Push the left hand into the wall for the leverage to twist to the left.
6. Using your arms and legs strongly, carefully create the power for a deep twist of the spine. Look over your left shoulder. Move your right ribs, not your shoulder, toward the wall. Retain a vertically elongated spine; do not tilt your head.
7. Root down through your right sitting bone to stabilize the base of the pose while turning to the left.

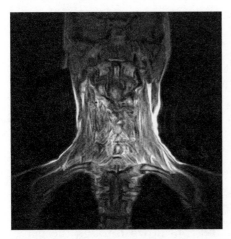
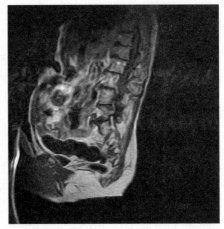

Figure 33. *Paraspinal muscles stimulate almost every imaginable aspect of the cervical vertebrae (left), yet the lumbar spine stays remarkably vertical and safe, even in a 90-degree twist like Ardha Matsyendrasana (right).*

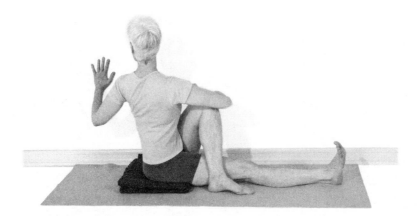

8. Continue to breathe and soften internally to receive the twist. There may be a subtle inner turn still possible even when your spine and ribs seem to have reached their limit.

9. After several breaths, return to face your knees and uncross your legs.

10. Repeat all actions above on the second side.

11. After doing both sides, sit for a moment to feel the effects of this pose, which does its work in so many areas of the body.

PREVENTION VARIATION

1. Place a folded blanket on your mat and sit on the blanket with your legs stretched out in front of you.
2. Manually widen your buttocks and thighs (see pages 87–88). This will help you avoid a slumped posture. Your sitting bones move back and apart.
3. Bend your right knee and bring the foot under your left leg to the outside of your left hip, the knee on the floor and pointing forward. Bend the left knee and place the left foot on the floor to the outside of your right leg, with the shin vertical. Place both hands on your left knee.
4. As you inhale, lift your spine up and root down through the pelvic bones. Isometrically widen your thighs, even though they will not move. This action will help your spine to lengthen up for the twist. It also pulls strongly on the pelvic bones and trochanters.

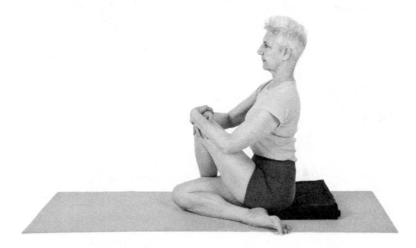

5. As you exhale, firm your abdominal muscles, lengthen your tailbone down, and turn toward the left. Cross your right elbow to the outside of your left knee and point the hand upward.
6. Bring your left hand to the floor behind you and pause to breathe.

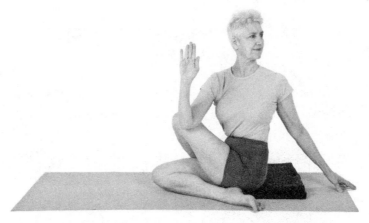

7. As you inhale, become taller. As you exhale, twist more.

8. Look over your left shoulder. Retain a vertically elongated spine; do not tilt your head.

9. Root down through both sides of the pelvis to stabilize the base of the pose.

10. Continue to breathe and soften internally to receive the twist. There may be a subtle inner turn still possible even when your spine and ribs appear to have reached their limit.

11. After several breaths, return to face your knees. Uncross your legs and stretch them straight in front of you.

12. Repeat all actions on the second side.

13. After completing both sides, sit for a moment to feel the effects of this pose, which does its work in many areas of the body.

A more intense version of this pose wraps the arms around the raised bent leg. Follow the steps above to prepare, then wrap the arms without forcing in the shoulders.

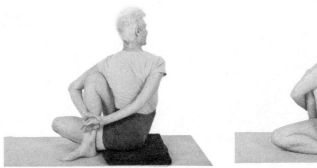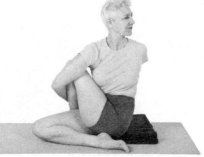

10. EKA PADA RAJAKAPOTASANA
Pigeon Pose

Purpose: Stimulates all aspects of the femur, pelvis, torso, and neck. Also improves hip extension and external rotation, which in turn improve balance.

Avoiding pitfalls: Face your hips squarely forward even though the legs are moving in separate directions in the pose. Move into the pose gradually.

OSTEOPOROSIS VARIATION

Contraindications: Total hip replacement.

Props: A chair, an optional blanket, and a table.

1. Place the chair facing the table and sit sideways on the front edge of the chair, with your left side toward the table. Rest your left forearm on the table, your right forearm on the chair back. You can sit on a blanket for comfort, or to raise the height of your pelvis.

2. Turn your right knee out to the side and place your right heel up, toes on the floor. Alternatively, if there is a rung on your chair, your foot can be up on it.

3. Keep your pelvis facing squarely forward (perpendicular to the side of

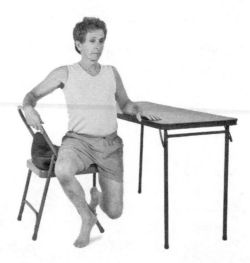

the table) and carefully slide your left foot back on the floor. You can lean forward a bit to enable the leg to reach back.

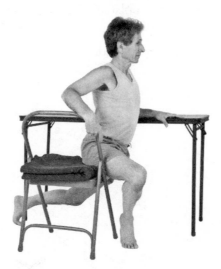

4. Firm your leg muscles. Isometrically abduct your upper legs away from the midline.
5. Curl your tailbone down and lift your abdomen up.
6. Remaining steady in the pelvis, extend the left leg back. The back knee can be bent, but straighten it as much as possible. Lift up through your spine.
7. This pose creates a strong stretch in the hips when the backward action of one leg and the lift of the spine are balanced. Push into the table and chair with your arms to lift the spine more.
8. Breathe fully as you continue the actions for 30 to 60 seconds, then release.
9. Repeat on the second side.

OSTEOPENIA VARIATION

Contraindications: Prepatellar bursitis, spinal stenosis, recent abdominal surgery, abdominal and ventral hernias, facet syndrome (segmental rigidity), total hip replacement, spondylolisthesis.
Props: A yoga mat, a chair, a bolster, and possibly a blanket.

1. Place a bolster 12 to 16 inches from the front of a chair on your yoga mat. Add a folded blanket under the bolster if your hips are stiff.

2. Position yourself onto the bolster, your right leg in front, left leg behind.

3. Bend your right knee out to the side.

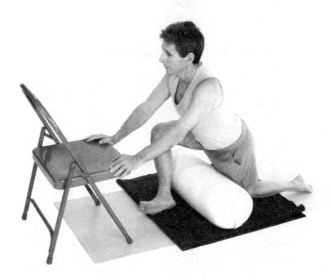

4. Stretch your left leg straight back, kneecap and toenails facing down. Alternatively, you can tuck the back toes under.

5. Lean with your arms on the chair for support.

6. Check that your pelvis is facing straight forward. Pull your left hip forward if necessary.

7. Firm your leg muscles and isometrically abduct your upper thighs away from the midline.

8. Curl your tailbone down and lift your abdomen up.

9. Without turning your pelvis, settle it down as much as possible; slide the back leg back farther if you can.

10. Stretch out through the back leg and up through your entire spine. Continue to face the chair directly.

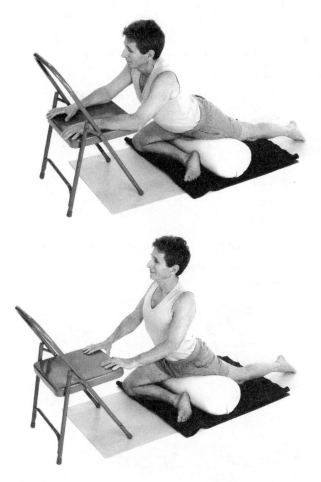

11. Remain poised in the midline for this asymmetrical pose during several quiet breaths, then release.

12. Repeat on the second side.

PREVENTION VARIATION

Contraindications: Prepatellar bursitis, hamstring tear, spinal stenosis, recent abdominal surgery, hernias, facet syndrome (segmental rigidity), total hip replacement, spondylolisthesis.

Props: A yoga mat and a rolled blanket.

Avoiding pitfalls: Face your hips squarely forward, your front leg open to the side, back leg straight behind you.

1. Roll up a blanket and place it on the mat. Position yourself on the rolled blanket with your right leg in front, left leg behind.
2. Bend your right knee out to the side.
3. Stretch your left leg straight back, kneecap facing down, toes tucked under.
4. Support your upper body with your hands on the floor on either side of your front knee.
5. Check that your pelvis is facing straight forward. Rotate your left hip forward if necessary.
6. Firm your leg muscles.
7. Isometrically abduct your upper thighs away from the midline.
8. Curl your tailbone down and lift your abdomen up.

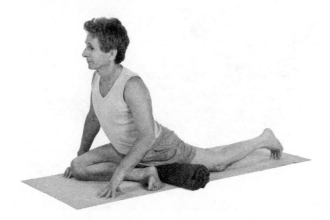

9. Without turning your pelvis, settle it down as much as possible; slide the back leg back farther if you can. Leaning forward will help you to do this.
10. Stretch out through the back leg. Rise up through your entire spine with your shoulders back. Turn your lower torso to the right enough to remain facing straight forward.
11. Remain poised in the midline for this asymmetrical pose for several breaths, then release.

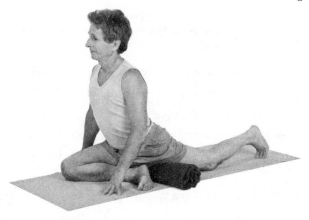

12. Repeat on the second side.

There are three more good ways to practice this pose for prevention. Follow all preparations in the variations above if you want to try these.

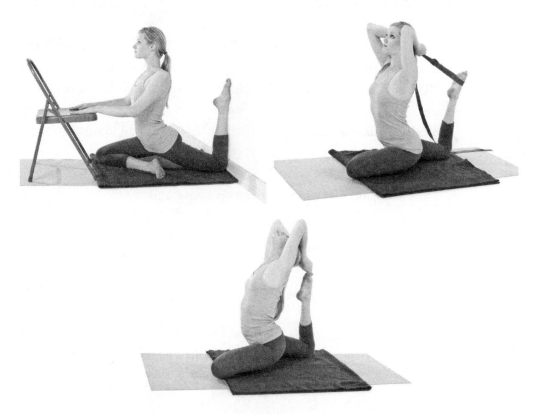

11. BALASANA   Child's Pose

Purpose: To stimulate the anterior lumbar vertebral bodies in flexion, the posterior thoracic vertebral bodies in extension, and to flex the hips as a counter-pose to backbends.

Avoiding pitfalls: Use the support of the props (if called for) to create a comfortable pose. Extend the spine forward as much as possible.

OSTEOPOROSIS VARIATION

Contraindications: (absolute) vertebral fracture; (relative) colostomy, prepatellar bursitis, meniscal tear, cruciate ligament tear, severe arthritis of the knee.

Props: A yoga mat, two or three blankets, and a chair.

1. Come onto your hands and knees on a stack of one or two folded blankets. Place the chair in front of you.
2. Position yourself with your feet half on and half off the edge of the blankets. This will moderate the stretch on your feet and ankles. Place the other folded blanket in the fold at the back of your knees to reduce possible strain there.
3. Widen your knees apart, about six inches more than hip-width.
4. Fold your hips back toward your heels.
5. Reach forward with your chest, stack one hand on the other on the chair seat, and rest your forehead on your hands.

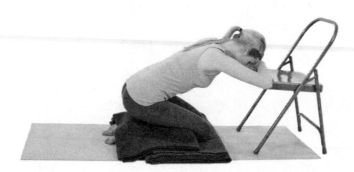

6. Breathe deeply. Reduce effort and surrender tension in your body and mind. When you are ready, come out of the pose by lifting your head and sitting up. Use your arms for support.

OSTEOPENIA VARIATION

Contraindications: Knee pain.

Props: A yoga mat, a blanket, and a block.

Avoiding pitfalls: Extend the thoracic spine as you move into the pose.

1. Come onto your hands and knees on a folded blanket.
2. Widen your knees apart, about six inches more than hip-width.
3. Stretch and spread your toes.
4. Place the block in front of you. Fold your hips back toward your heels.
5. Reach forward with your chest and rest your forehead on the block. Place your forearms on the mat on either side of the block.

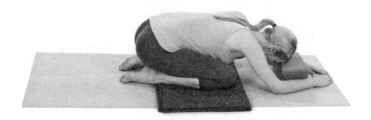

6. Breathe deeply. Reduce effort and surrender tension in your body and mind. When you are ready, come out of the pose by lifting your head and sitting up.

PREVENTION VARIATION

Contraindication: Knee pain.

Props: A yoga mat and one blanket.

Avoiding pitfalls: Be careful to extend the thoracic spine.

1. Come onto your hands and knees on a folded blanket.
2. Widen your knees apart, about six inches more than hip-width.
3. Stretch and spread your toes.

4. Fold your hips back toward your heels.

5. Reach forward with your chest and rest your forehead on your folded hands, or on the floor with your arms stretching forward.

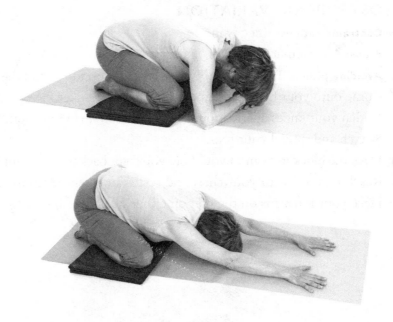

6. Breathe deeply. Reduce effort and surrender tension in your body and mind. When you are ready, come out of the pose by lifting your head and sitting up.

12. SAVASANA   Corpse Pose

Purpose: To cease effort, relax, assimilate, and consolidate gains.

Contraindications: Late pregnancy.

Props: A yoga mat, three blankets, optional eye cover.

Avoiding pitfalls: After the initial setup, avoid fussing and fidgeting, become settled. B. K. S. Iyengar commented in *Light on Yoga*, "By remaining motionless for some time and keeping the mind still while you are fully conscious, you learn to relax. This conscious relaxation invigorates and refreshes both body and mind. But it is much harder to keep the mind than the body still. Therefore, this apparently easy posture is one of the most difficult to master."

1. Make sure the space is quiet and safe from distractions.

2. Fold one blanket to support a slight arch of your thoracic spine, roll the second for under your knees, and fold the third one to support your neck and head. An eye cover may help to relax your face and allow you to retreat from all outer stimuli.

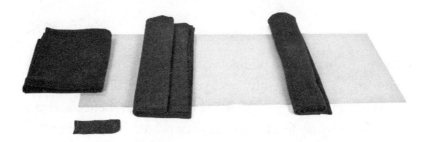

3. Lie on your back with arms at your sides, palms up. Make sure that the chest-supporting blanket allows your shoulders to be flat on the floor. Refold or adjust as necessary.

4. Adjust your hips by turning your legs inward to widen the back of the pelvis, then let the feet roll apart as you relax.

5. Lengthen your buttocks away from the waist if you feel any compression in your lower back.

6. Tuck your shoulder blades gently in toward the spine to open the front of your chest.

7. Make sure that your neck is long and your chin and forehead are level. Then guide your attention through your whole body systematically from head to toe and back again, letting each part relax thoroughly.

8. Do not fret if your mind produces thoughts; just watch them unemotionally without being drawn into the content. Be a compassionate witness. You might notice yourself reviewing an event, thinking of a person, or making a plan. Try not to follow the pull of any thoughts, but passively observe them come and go. Trust in the process of letting go.

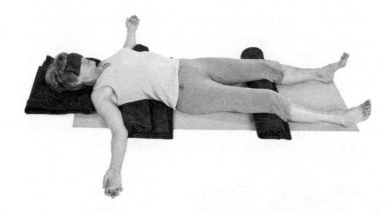

9. After 5 to 10 minutes of quiet rest, take a few deeper breaths, stretch your arms and legs gently, bend your knees, then softly roll to the side. Take your time getting up, and respect whatever effects, changes, and benefits you may feel from your yoga practice. Remember your intention. Affirm your process of growth and healing.

Poses That Focus on Balance

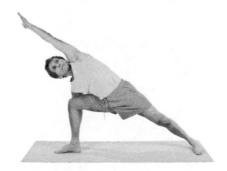

1. UTTHITA PARSVAKONASANA
Side Angle Pose

Purpose: Produces stimulating torque to the entire central and peripheral skeleton.

Contraindications: Ischial bursitis, coccygodynia, intervertebral disc herniation, spinal vertebral fracture, labral tear of shoulder or hip, carpal tunnel syndrome.

Props: A yoga mat and a chair, possibly a blanket or block.

Avoiding pitfalls: Adjust for your height as necessary. If your front foot doesn't reach the floor easily, place a block under it. If you are tall, put a folded blanket on the chair seat. Even though you have a chair for support, work diligently in the pose.

OSTEOPOROSIS VARIATION

1. Sit on a chair with your knees wide apart.
2. Manually widen your buttocks and upper thighs (see pages 87–88) to create the correct tilt of your pelvis and to free the hip joints.

3. Open your right knee out to the side and place your foot directly under the knee.

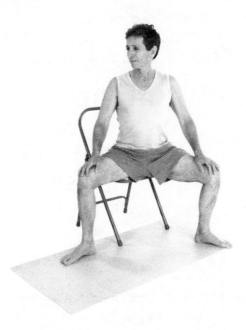

4. Lean to the right, moving from your hip, not your waist, and rest your right forearm on your thigh.
5. Move the left leg to the left until it stretches straight, keeping the toes and the knee facing forward. More of your weight will now be on your right hip.
6. With the muscles of your legs and abdomen active, curl your tailbone diagonally down toward your left foot, along the same angle at which your whole body is now inclined.
7. Firm your abdominal muscles and from the core of your pelvis extend out into both legs and up through your spine.
8. Place your left hand on your left hip and roll your left shoulder back until your entire upper body faces outward.
9. For more intensity, turn your torso enough to the left to grasp the back of the chair with your left hand, and look up.

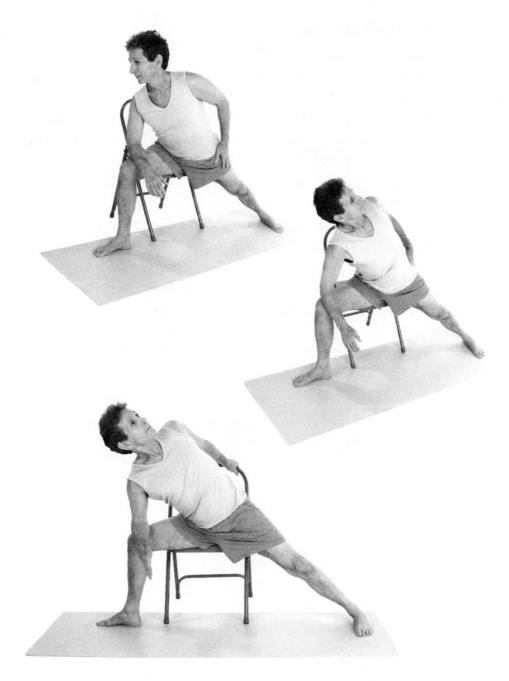

10. Hold the pose for several quiet breaths, and then release.
11. Repeat on the second side.

OSTEOPENIA VARIATION

Props: A yoga mat and a wall.

Avoiding pitfalls: Maintain full strength in the back leg, and align the front bent knee carefully toward the second toe.

1. Place your mat alongside a wall. Stand with your back to the wall and step your feet apart so that your ankles line up under your wrists when your arms are stretched to the sides.

2. Turn the right foot and leg parallel to the wall, but don't turn your torso. Your left foot faces straight out from the wall.

3. Inhale, firm your legs and lengthen up through the spine. As you exhale, bend your right knee until it is over the ankle. Point the knee toward the second toe.

4. As you inhale again, incline your torso over your right hip and rest your right forearm on your thigh. Your left hand can rest on your hip.

5. Anchor your left foot. Move your left thigh back toward the wall, revolving the entire thigh slightly inward at first, toward the midline.

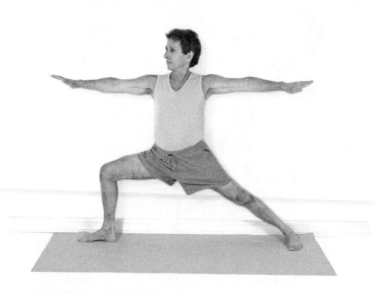

6. Curl your tailbone toward the left heel, tighten your lower belly, and now rotate your left knee outward to face away from the wall. These actions will increase your power and stability.

7. Roll your left shoulder and chest up toward the ceiling without disturbing the alignment of your legs. Stretch your left arm straight out from your shoulder.

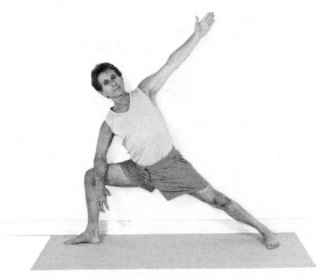

8. From the pelvis, the center of the pose, stretch in all directions, pulling your shoulders back toward the wall.

9. Hold for several quiet breaths, noticing the balance of strength and expansion in this exhilarating pose.

10. Inhale as you come back up.

11. Repeat on the second side.

PREVENTION VARIATION

Props: A yoga mat and a block.

1. Place a block toward the right side of your mat.

2. Step your feet apart so that your ankles line up under your wrists when your arms are stretched to the sides.

3. Turn the right foot and knee parallel to the long edge of the mat, but

don't turn your torso. Place your right foot so that the block is on the big-toe side of the foot.

4. Inhale, firm your legs, and lengthen up through the spine. As you exhale, bend your right knee until it is over the ankle. Point the knee toward the second toe.

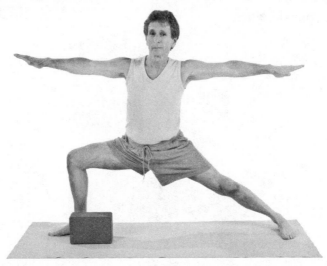

5. On your next exhalation, bend your torso to the right and place your right forearm on your right thigh. Place your left hand on your waist.

6. Anchor the left foot. Move your left thigh back, revolving the entire thigh slightly inward at first, toward the midline.

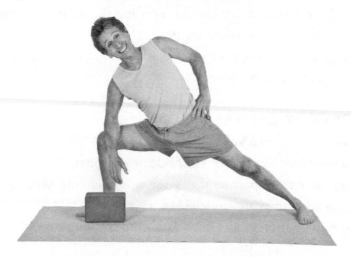

7. Curl your tailbone toward your left heel, tighten your lower belly, and now rotate your left knee outward to face straight ahead. These actions increase your control and stability.

8. Place your right hand on the block and raise your left arm straight up toward the ceiling.

9. Pause for a breath to check: Are your legs fully engaged with muscular strength? Is your left leg back enough to be in the same line with the rest of your body, not pushing forward? Is your abdomen firm? Are your arms pulled into the shoulders?

10. Bring your left arm over your ear, palm facing down. Bring the arm into the same diagonal line as the rest of the body, not forward or back.

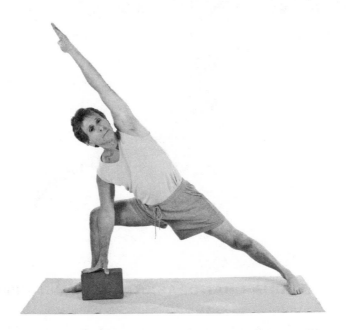

11. From the pelvis, the center of the pose, stretch in all directions.

12. Hold for several quiet breaths, observing the balance of strength and expansion in this vigorous and exhilarating pose.

13. Inhale as you come back up.

14. Repeat on the second side.

The full classic pose: Enter the pose as instructed in steps 2 through 7. One hand goes to the floor behind the foot of the bent leg, the other arm stretches overhead. Follow steps 9 through 14 above.

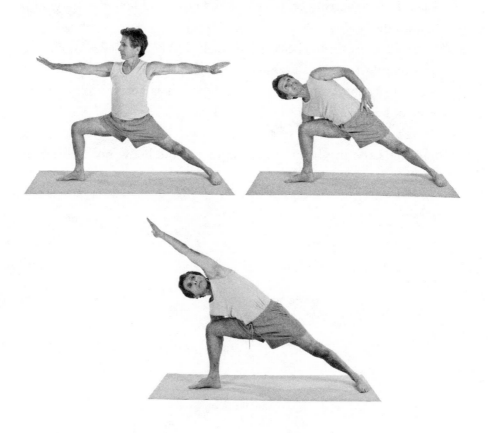

2. ARDHA CHANDRASANA   Half Moon Pose

Purpose: To refine balance; laterally load the lumbar, thoracic, and cervical vertebrae, iliac bones, inner and outer femur; generate forces on the wrists, arms, and shoulders; and improve balance.

Contraindications: Imbalance, plantar fasciitis, vertebral fracture, Hill-Sachs deformity, subscapularis bursitis/tendonitis, subdeltoid bursitis, carpal tunnel syndrome.

Props: A yoga mat, a wall, a chair, and a block.

Avoiding pitfalls: Do not rush this pose; carefully and deliberately progress from one position to the next.

OSTEOPOROSIS VARIATION

1. Place your mat alongside a wall and a chair to the left side, facing toward you. With your back to the wall, place your right foot close to the front of the chair and turn the foot parallel to the wall. Inhale and expand from inside.

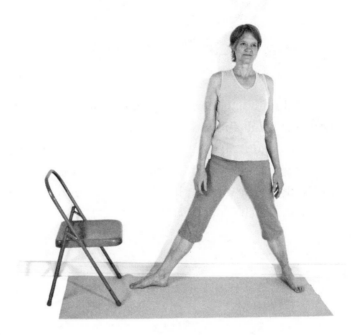

2. Bend your right knee; check that the knee points over the toes. Position your right hip lightly against the wall to stabilize your balance.
3. Place your right hand on the chair seat. Lightly touch the floor with the toes of your left foot while you establish your balance on your right leg. Rest your left hand on your hip.
4. Inhale as you firm the muscles of your legs. Roll your left shoulder back to align your torso with the wall. Look down at the chair to help

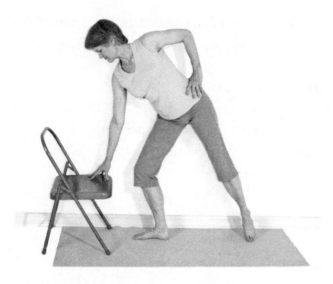

balance, but avoid slumping your body; simply turn your head, keeping your shoulders parallel to the wall.

5. On your next inhalation, lift your left leg off the floor and stretch it
   back behind you along the wall. Most of your weight is now on your
   right leg, with only a little on your hand. The picture shows an added
   block on the chair, which is optional.

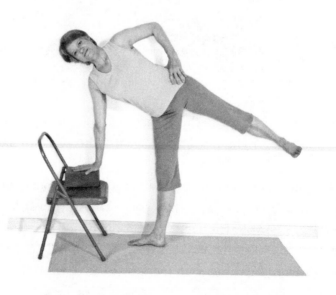

6. Use the leg muscles strongly and stretch through your heels.

7. Breathing fully and smoothly, expand out from your pelvis in all directions. Touch the wall with your back as necessary for balance.

8. To come down, stretch back through your left leg as you bring your left foot to the floor, then bring your upper body to vertical.

9. Repeat on the second side.

OSTEOPENIA VARIATION

1. Place your mat alongside a wall and the block to the side, next to the wall. Stand with your back to the wall and place your right foot about 12 to 18 inches from the block. Turn the right foot parallel to the wall.

2. Bend your right knee and check that the knee points over the toes. Rest your right hip lightly against the wall to stabilize your balance.

3. Reach your right hand to the block; lift the left heel off the floor. Lightly touch the floor with the toes of your left foot while you establish your balance on your right leg. Your left hand rests on your hip.

4. Inhale, firm the muscles of your legs, and roll your left shoulder back to align it with the wall. Look down at the floor to help you balance (not pictured), but avoid slumping your body; simply turn your head to the right, keeping your shoulders parallel to the wall.

5. On your next inhalation, lift your left leg off the floor and stretch it back behind you along the wall and parallel to the floor. Use the leg muscles strongly and stretch through your heels. Bring the left hip up and back toward the wall to stack over the right hip. This action requires that the right leg be very steady.

6. Stretch the standing leg straight with a strong squeezing action of the muscles just above your knee.

7. Breathing fully and smoothly, stretch your left arm up straight near the wall. Expand out in all directions from the core of your pelvis. Find your balance with the wall as a directional reference but avoid touching it if possible.

8. Look straight out from the wall, extending your neck long.

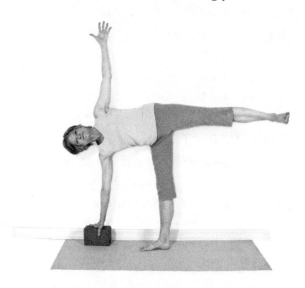

9. To come down, stretch back through your left leg, bring your left foot to the floor, and bring your upper body to vertical.
10. Repeat on the second side.

PREVENTION VARIATION

1. Place a chair on the right end of your mat, facing toward you. Place your right foot about 10 inches in front of the chair, pointing directly toward it, and stretch your arms to the sides.

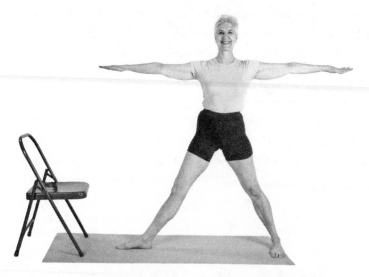

2. Bend your right knee and check that it points over the toes. Tuck your right hip under you to stabilize your balance.

3. Place your right forearm on the seat of the chair. Lightly touch the floor with the toes of your left foot while you establish your balance on your right leg. Rest your left hand on your hip.

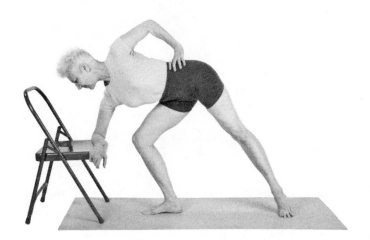

4. Inhale as you firm the muscles of your legs. Roll your left shoulder back slowly to align your torso over your right leg and foot. Look down at the chair to help your balance, but avoid slumping your body; simply turn your head to the right, keeping your shoulders perpendicular to the floor.

5. On your next inhalation, lift your left leg and stretch it back behind you, parallel to the floor. Use the leg muscles strongly and stretch through your heel.

6. Lift the left hip up and back to stack it over the right hip. This action requires that the right leg be very steady.

7. Stretch the right leg as straight as possible, with a strong squeezing action of the muscles just above your knee.

8. Breathing fully and smoothly, stretch your left arm vertically. Expand out in all directions from the core of your pelvis.

9. Look straight out or down, lengthening your neck.

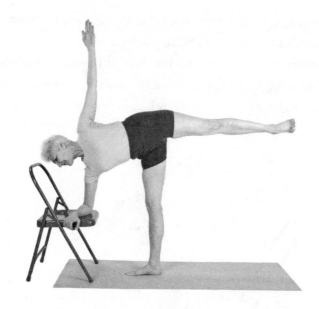

10. To come down, stretch back through your left leg and bring your left foot to the floor, then bring your upper body to vertical.

11. Repeat on the second side.

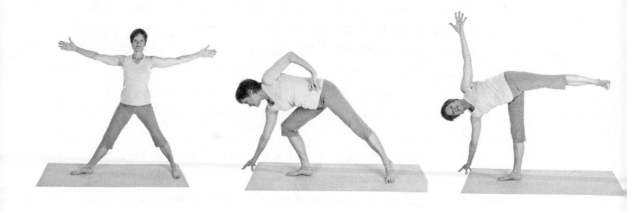

These pictures show how to enter the full pose unsupported. Follow the preparatory steps outlined to align your whole body in one plane.

3. VIRABHADRASANA I   Upright Lunge

Purpose: To stress the thigh and pelvic bones with hip extension, to stimulate lumbar and thoracic vertebral bodies, and to promote balance.

Contraindications: Hyperlordosis, spondylolisthesis, spondylolysis, anterior cruciate sprain.

OSTEOPOROSIS VARIATION

Props: A yoga mat, a chair, and an optional blanket or block.

Avoiding pitfalls: Even though you are sitting on the chair, engage your muscles fully.

1. Sit sideways on the front edge of a chair with your left hip and leg off the chair. Use a blanket under your hips if you are tall.

2. Position your right foot directly under the right knee, facing directly forward over the toes. If you are smaller and your front foot does not easily reach the floor, place a block under that foot.

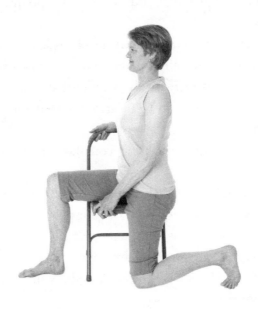

3. Slide your left leg back a bit and lean forward slightly, placing one hand on the chair back and one on the seat.

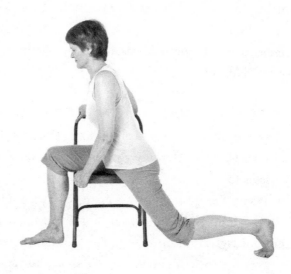

4. Inhale and stretch up through your spine from the inside. Pull your shoulders back.

5. Firm your leg muscles and isometrically broaden your thighs and buttocks. Lift your inner belly up and lengthen down through your tailbone. These actions increase the stimuli that will strengthen the bones, as well as prepare you to balance without the chair in later variations of the pose.

6. Maintain these actions as you bring your head and shoulders back over your hips.

7. Stretch your left leg back farther. Bring your left hand to your hip to secure the forward-facing alignment of your pelvis.

8. Lift your arms out to the side and then up near your ears.

9. Stretch up through your spine and arms with full power. Work your legs as though you did not have the chair under you. You can prepare to lift off without really doing so.

10. Exhale and release your arms down.

11. Repeat on the second side.

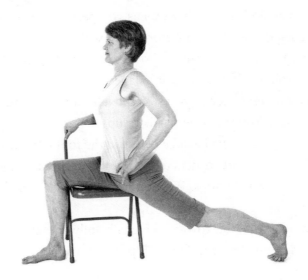

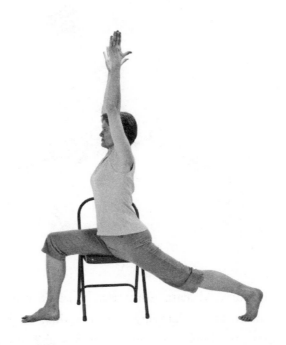

OSTEOPENIA VARIATION

Props: A yoga mat and a chair.

Avoiding pitfalls: Set the pelvis carefully, squarely facing the back of the chair, and keep it that way as you perform the pose. Don't let the back leg droop. Align the front knee with the second toe.

1. Place a chair at one end of your mat. Stand facing the back of your chair and lightly touch it for balance.

2. Bend the right knee as you step the left foot back until your right shin is vertical. Your back heel will be up.

3. Attentively find the balance between the four corners of the right foot and the two front corners of the left foot. Point the right knee straight forward over the toes. Position the back heel over the center of the toes.

4. Lean forward a bit toward the chair, fully stretch your back leg, and firm the muscles from feet to hips.

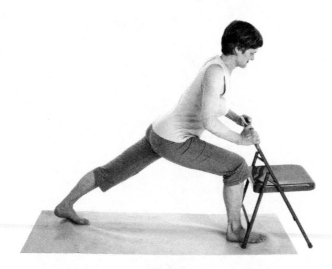

5. Retain the forward lean, isometrically widen the upper thighs and pelvic bones without changing your feet, then lengthen your tailbone down. Draw the lower belly in and up to stabilize your pelvis.

6. Bring your torso upright and retract your shoulders back until they are just above your hips.

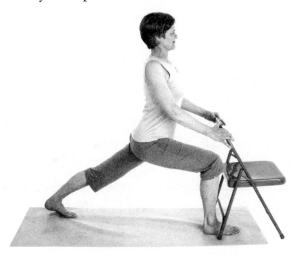

7. If and when you feel steady, let go of the chair and stretch your arms up alongside your ears.
8. Remain poised in this strong lunge with full attention. Expand out from the pelvis through your legs, spine, and arms, fully engaging the body.
9. Repeat on the second side.

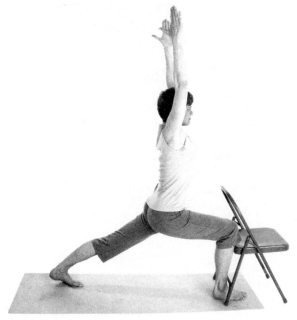

PREVENTION VARIATION

With the back heel down on the second mat, there is a longer overall stretch than in the osteopenia variation.

Props: Two yoga mats and a chair.

Avoiding pitfalls: See osteopenia variation.

1. Place a chair at one end of your mat. Stand facing the back of your chair and lightly touch it for balance.
2. Step your left foot back until your right shin is vertical, knee over the ankle. Place the folded mat under your heel (the mat will best support you if angled as shown).
3. Attentively find the balance between the four corners of both feet, and point the right knee straight forward over the toes. The back foot and knee are slightly turned to the left without changing the alignment of the pelvis.

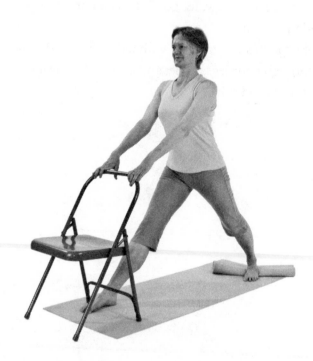

4. Lean forward toward the chair, fully stretch your back leg, and firm the muscles from feet to hips.

5. Retain the forward lean, widen the upper thighs and pelvic bones without changing your feet, then lengthen your tailbone down and draw the lower belly in and up to stabilize your pelvis.

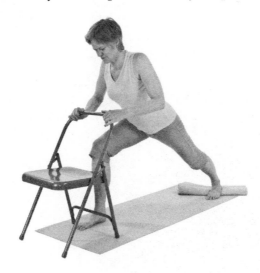

6. Bring your torso upright and retract your shoulders back until they are just above your hips. Spread your arms wide and lift your spine.

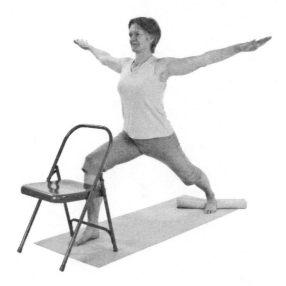

7. When you feel steady, stretch your arms up near your ears. Look
   straight ahead. Breathe fully and confidently as you maintain this
   pose. Expand out from the pelvis through your legs, spine, and arms,
   fully engaging the body.

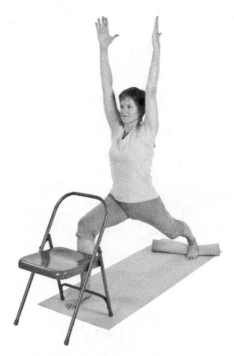

8. Repeat on the second side.

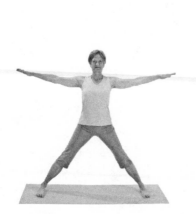 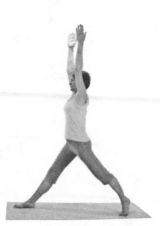 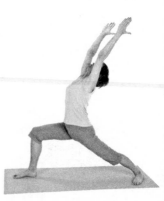

The full pose contains all the above elements, plus the spine arches, the arms reach back, and the back heel is on the floor, requiring more ankle stretch. A balance of muscular strength pulling in and expansion stretching out will help you to maintain stability in this dynamic pose. Make one long continuous span from your back foot to your fingertips. This pose requires tremendous strength, flexibility, and balance. Remain soft and open as you stretch. Do not force, but explore and radiate both forward and outward.

4. PARIVRTTA PARSVAKONASANA
Revolved Side Angle Pose

Purpose: To oppose the arm and shoulder with contralateral pelvis, hip, and leg muscles, increasing forces applied to both, and to expose lumbar, thoracic, and cervical vertebrae to extreme torque. The entire spine revolves, creating resistive stress on the vertebrae, shoulders, and pelvic bones.

Contraindications: *For all variations*, ischial bursitis, coccygodynia. *For osteopenia and prevention variations*, Hill-Sachs deformity, repeated shoulder subluxation, imbalance, plantar fasciitis, anterior cruciate tear, patellofemoral arthralgia, Dupuytren's contracture, intervertebral disc herniation, spinal vertebral fracture, labral tear, hamstring sprain, carpal tunnel syndrome, total hip replacement, scoliosis, herniated lumbar disc, previous lumbar surgery, moderate or severe rotatory scoliosis.

Props: A yoga mat, a blanket, a chair, and a wall.

Avoiding pitfalls: Proceed carefully in each phase of the pose to maintain balance. Keep the hips square to the front and hug the midline. Don't hold your breath.

OSTEOPOROSIS VARIATION

1. Place a chair on your mat. Sit sideways with your left hip on the front of the seat. If you are tall, sit on a folded blanket. Place your left foot

directly under your knee. Hang your right thigh down alongside the chair, but keep your pelvis level.

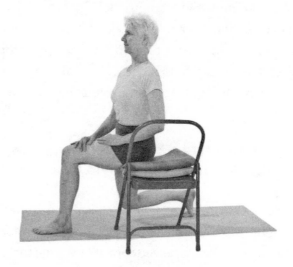

2. Inhale and lift your spine, firming the muscles and expanding your torso from inside. Stretch your right leg back behind you. Hold the chair back with your left hand and rest your right hand on your left thigh.

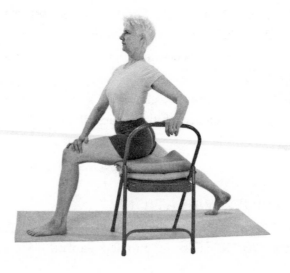

3. Exhale and bend forward. Place your right forearm on your left thigh and turn toward the back of the chair. Hold the chair with both hands.

4. Hug in toward the midline and revolve your spine around its axis, starting at the lower back and lower belly and working up. Your pelvis stays stable on the chair, your legs steady, your back straight.

5. Roll your left shoulder back and extend through your neck, looking to the left.

6. Hold the pose for several breaths with steady strength and maximum length in your spine.

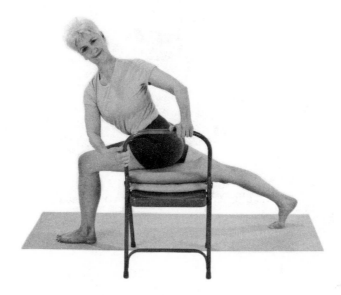

7. Untwist to face forward again and bring your right leg forward next to your left leg.

8. Sit sideways on the right hip to repeat on the second side.

9. After the second side, sit on the chair facing forward to rest and breathe quietly.

OSTEOPENIA VARIATION

1. Place your mat along a wall and a blanket on the middle of the mat.

2. Kneel with your left side toward the wall. Step your left foot forward,

aligned under the knee. Leave 4 to 6 inches between yourself and the wall.

3. Inhale, expand on the inside, and firm your leg muscles for stability before twisting. The pelvis remains aligned straight ahead.

4. Exhale and turn toward the wall. Twist your spine to the left while

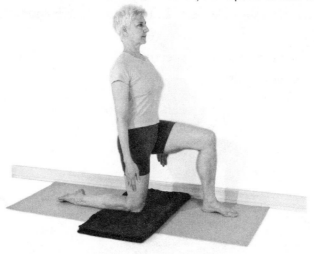

the pelvis remains aligned perpendicular to the wall. Do not let your back hunch forward.

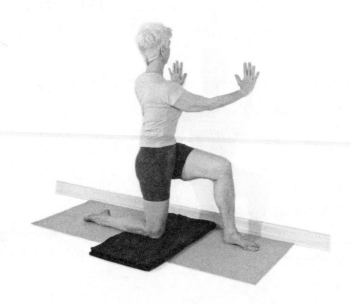

5. Bend forward to bring your right elbow to the top or outside of your left knee. Touch the wall with both hands.

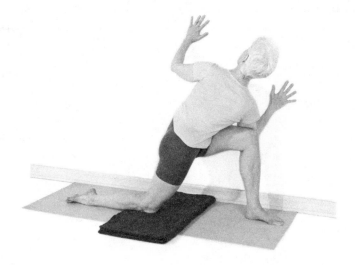

6. Hug in toward the midline and revolve your spine around its axis, starting at the lower back and lower belly and moving up. Your pelvis and your legs remain firm and steady.
7. Roll your left shoulder back and extend through your neck, looking to the left.
8. To intensify the pose, tuck your back foot's toes under and stretch that leg straight back, lifting the knee off the floor, while continuing to twist (not pictured). Hold the pose for several calm breaths, with steady strength and maximum length in your spine.
9. Untwist to face forward again.
10. Turn to bring your right side toward the wall with your right leg forward, left leg back and twist to the right toward the wall.
11. After the second side, sit or stand normally to rest.

PREVENTION VARIATION

1. Place a folded blanket on your mat. Come onto your hands and knees with the blanket under your knees.

2. Step your left foot forward between your hands. Move your right knee back a few inches.

3. Raise your upper body to vertical. Place your hands on your hips.

4. Inhale, firm your leg muscles to stabilize the legs, and lift up your torso.

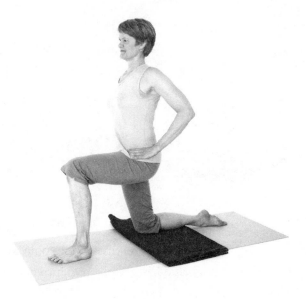

5. Exhale, incline your entire torso forward, twist to the left, and place your right elbow outside the left knee.

6. Pull your left hip crease back with your left hand.

7. For the next few breaths lengthen the spine with each inhalation, and twist more to the left as you exhale. Lead the twisting action with your back right ribs, and move into the pose more deeply with each exhalation.

8. Open your chest. Hold your head in line with the spine as much as possible. A combination of strength to maintain the actions and softness to maintain the breath are important here.

9. Tuck the back foot's toes under and raise the back knee. Straighten the back leg and draw every part of your body in toward the midline. Remain aligned from your head to your back heel and extend through the top of your head.

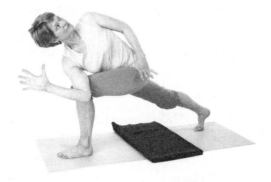

10. Remain poised and twisting with full commitment and confidence.
11. To release, turn toward your front foot, step back with your front leg and rest in Child's Pose.
12. Repeat on the second side.

For the full pose, all you have to add is the arm position and lower the back heel to the floor.

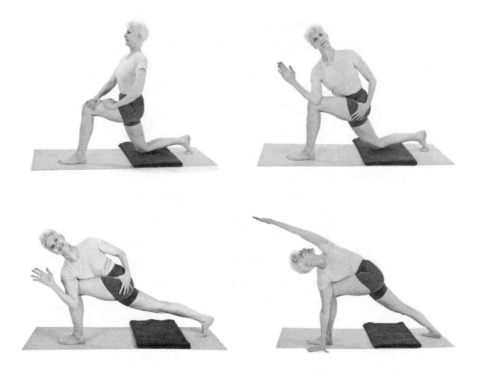

5. VASISTHASANA   Side Inclined Balance

Purpose: To apply force asymmetrically to the ribs, the lateral aspects of all the vertebral bodies, and the pelvic bones. To apply compressive asymmetrical forces at the wrists, arms, and shoulders, stimulating osteoblasts and osteocytes at all locations. To develop balance.

Contraindications: *For all these variations*, profound weakness, Hill-Sachs deformity, Bankart fracture, shoulder subluxation, trochanteric bursitis, lateral collateral ligamentous laxity. If scoliosis is present, perform this pose only on the convex side of the thoracolumbar curve. *For osteopenia and prevention variations*, Dupuytren's contracture, carpal tunnel syndrome, fifth metatarsal fracture.

Props: A yoga mat, a wall, and a chair.

Avoiding pitfalls: Pull your upper arm and shoulder back before putting weight on them. Line your head up with your spine. Don't be tentative; be firm and expansive with your whole body.

OSTEOPOROSIS VARIATION

1. Place your mat alongside a wall and a chair facing toward the mat and the wall.
2. Lie on your left side with your back to the wall. Raise your torso up enough to place your left forearm on the floor perpendicular to the wall.
3. Bend your knees. Pull your shoulders back to align your upper body parallel to the wall. Align your head with your spine.
4. Place your right hand on the chair seat for support.
5. Inhaling, firm your abdominal muscles and your arms. Pull your back muscles in toward the spine.
6. Exhaling and maintaining the muscular firmness, lift your ribs up away from the floor. Your hips and legs remain on the floor. Press down on the chair as needed.

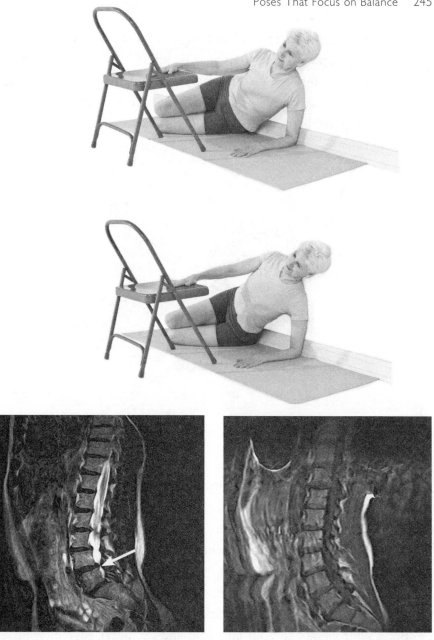

Figure 34. *Note that the spondylolisthesis (left) does not appear in the image on the right. The forces brought to bear on the anterior, posterior, and lateral spine in Vasisthasana reduce spondylolisthesis significantly. This demonstrates two points: Yoga can improve spinal alignment, and muscles attaching to the vertebrae can move them. Working to strengthen these muscles will apply the type of pressure on them that counters osteoporosis.*

7. Release down with your ribs, and prepare for the next stage.

8. Exhaling and maintaining muscular firmness, this time lift your hips up away from the floor. Your lower legs remain on the floor. Press down on the chair with your hand as needed. Lift your ribs enough to form a diagonal line from your left knee to your left shoulder

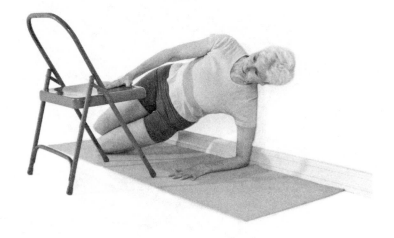

9. Maintain the pose as long as you can, then release.

10. Repeat on the second side.

OSTEOPENIA VARIATION

1. Place your mat alongside a wall.

2. Come onto your hands and knees with your left side near the wall. Move your knees back a few inches.

3. Take a deep breath.

4. Firm your arms, legs and spine, and lift your pelvis upward as much as possible into Downward Facing Dog as you exhale (see page 113).

5. Bring your weight to your left hand and the outer edge of your left foot. Place your right foot in front of the left foot. Firm and stretch the outer edges of both feet, pulling the little toes back.

6. Alternatively, step your right foot to the middle of the mat, pointing outward to help balance.

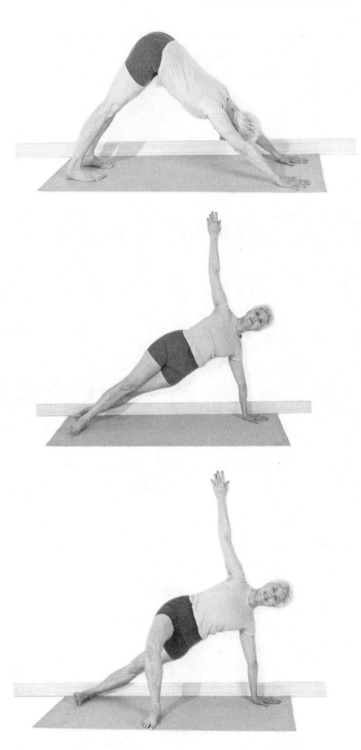

7. Stretch your right hand straight up. You can touch the wall with your back body for support if needed, or be near the wall without touching it in order to orient the back of your body accurately with the plane of the wall.

8. Lengthen your tailbone and pull your belly in and up, holding your body in one long line parallel to the wall.

9. Pull your shoulders back and look straight out from the wall. Align your head with your spine.

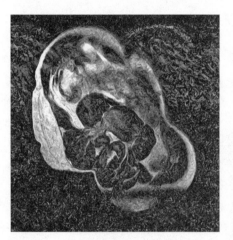 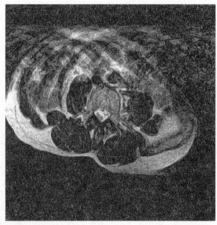

Figure 35. *Vasisthasana creates the large, light-colored diamond shaped spinal canal just below the horseshoe-shaped vertebra (right) from the truncated and irregular spinal canal, showing spinal stenosis (left). These MRI images were taken at the same spinal level 7 minutes apart.*

10. Exuberantly expand out from your center to your toes, fingertips, and the crown of your head.

11. Maintain the pose 20 to 30 seconds, then release.

12. Repeat on the second side.

PREVENTION VARIATION

1. Come onto your hands and knees. Move your knees back a few inches.

2. Take a deep breath in.

3. Firm your arms, legs, and spine, and lift up into Downward Facing Dog as you exhale.

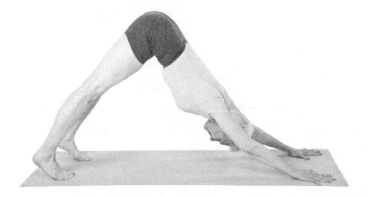

4. Bring your weight to your left hand and the outer edge of your left foot. Stack your right foot on top of your left. With both feet, firm and stretch the outer edges, pulling the little toes back.

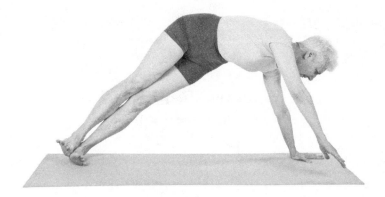

5. Stretch your right hand straight up. Pull your shoulders and thighs back.
6. Lengthen your tailbone and pull your belly in and up, making your body one long line from head to feet. Lift your pelvis and ribs away from the floor to create this long diagonal line, projecting out from the pelvis, out through your arms, legs, and spine.

7. Look either straight in front of you or up at the right hand.
8. Exuberantly charge the whole body and radiate in this pose.

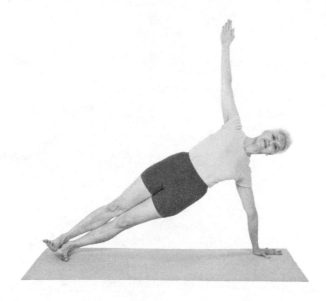

9. Maintain the pose as long as you can, then come down, placing both hands and feet on the floor for Downward- Facing Dog.
10. Repeat on the second side.

6. UPAVISTHA KONASANA
Wide Angle Seated Pose

Purpose: To apply bilateral leg stress from medial and lateral aspects and pressure to the pelvis and thoracolumbar spine.

Contraindications: Grade 3 or 4 anterior cruciate or meniscal tears, chondromalacia patellae, severe hip arthritis, sacroiliac joint derangement, herniated lumbar disc, ischial bursitis, profound weakness.

OSTEOPOROSIS VARIATION

Props: A yoga mat and a wall.

Avoiding pitfalls: Keep your knees facing out over your toes.

1. Place your yoga mat alongside a wall. Stand with your back to the wall, legs and feet turned out approximately 45 degrees to the side.
2. Inhale and lift your spine.
3. Bend your knees until your thighs are parallel to the floor, gradually moving your feet out from the wall as you do so. The knees should point the same direction as the toes.
4. Place your hands over the tops of your thighs, near the knees, with your fingers pointing outward.
5. Press your hands down to lift your spine up more, and curl your tailbone down. You can lean slightly forward if that feels right, but keep lifting your chest.

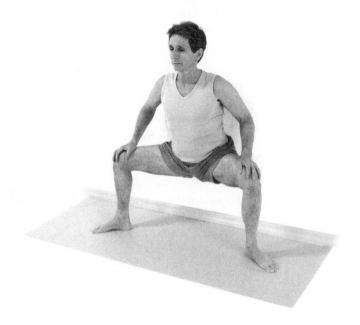

6. Widen your shoulders as you pull your elbows to your sides.
7. Hold with constant strength. Lengthen out from your pelvis through your thighs, and up through your entire torso.
8. When you're ready to come up, push down through your feet and straighten your legs, releasing your hands.

OSTEOPENIA VARIATION

Props: A yoga mat, one or two folded blankets, a chair, and optionally two towels.

Avoiding pitfalls: Use sufficient height under your hips so that you can tip the top of the pelvis forward. More height will accommodate tighter hamstrings.

1. Place a chair on your mat, facing in toward the middle of the mat. You will move it toward you once you are in the pose. Fold the blankets and place one corner facing the chair.
2. Sit on the front corner of the blankets with your legs 90 to 100 degrees apart.
3. Manually widen the backs of your thighs and your sitting bones, which will tip your pelvis forward at the top (see pages 87–88).
4. Place your hands on the chair seat. Align your legs with the kneecaps and toes pointing straight up. If your knees are more than an inch or so away from the floor, place a folded towel under each in order to feel a surface under your knees.
5. Inhaling, lift up through your spine and contract your leg muscles to fully straighten your knees. Push your thighs down as your lift your spine up.
6. Press down into the chair seat to increase the lift of your spine.

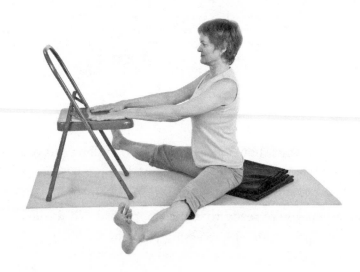

7. Tip your pelvis and spine forward as much as possible, hinging at the hips, not the waist. Maintain one long line from your pelvis to the crown of your head. Rest your forearms on the chair seat.

8. Firm and lift your abdomen and root down with your tailbone, keeping your spine long.

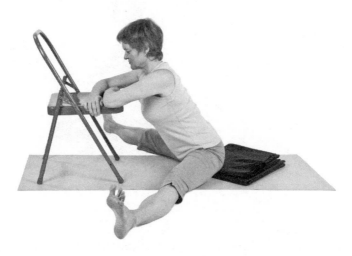

9. As you incline forward, maintain full strength in your leg muscles. The knees tend to pop up; continue to press them down.

10. Breathe quietly while holding the pose, then slowly release up to vertical.

PREVENTION VARIATION

Props: A yoga mat and a folded blanket.

Avoiding pitfalls: Avoid going farther forward than your hip flexibility allows. Root your legs down and extend the spine long, avoiding a rounded upper back.

1. Place a folded blanket on your mat. Sit on the front corner of the blanket with your legs spread 90 to 100 degrees apart.

2. Manually widen the back of your thighs and sitting bones, which will help your pelvis to tip forward at the top (see pages 87–88).

3. Place your fingertips beside your hips on the floor. Align your legs with the kneecaps and toes pointing straight up.

4. Inhaling, lift up through your spine and contract your quadriceps to fully straighten your knees. Push your thighs down as your lift your spine up.

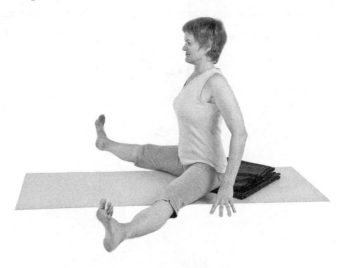

5. Press down with your fingertips on the floor to increase the lift of your spine.
6. Tip your pelvis and spine forward as much as possible, hinging at the hips, not the waist. Keep one long line from your pelvis to the crown of your head. Walk your hands out on the floor in front of you.
7. As your arms reach forward, pull your upper arms back into the shoulder sockets and lift your inner armpits up.

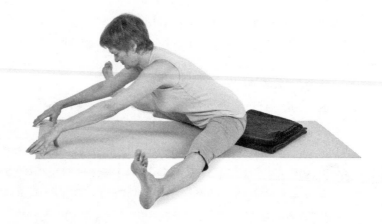

8. Firm and lift your abdomen and root down with your tailbone so that your lower spine stays long. Extend your head forward and up in line with your spine.

9. As you incline forward, maintain full strength in your leg muscles. The knees tend to pop up; continue to press them down.

10. Breathe quietly while holding the pose, then release up to vertical, maintaining the length in your spine.

In the full pose, be sure to balance the inward pull of the muscles with the expansion out through the straightened legs and long spine.

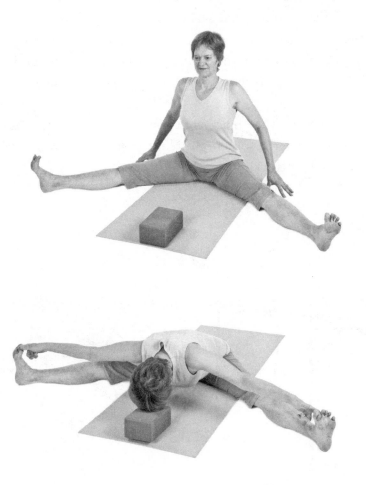

7. BADDHA KONASANA   Cobbler's Pose

Purpose: Exerts stimulating pressure on feet, ankles, calves, and thigh bones, lumbar and thoracic spine, and lateral pelvis.

Contraindications: Adductor tear, pubic separation, ischial bursitis, herniated lumbar disc.

Avoiding pitfalls: Maintain each action as you proceed to the next instruction.

OSTEOPOROSIS VARIATION

Props: A chair, a block, and a table.

1. Place a chair facing a table, and a block on the floor under the table.
2. Sit on the front edge of the chair and manually adjust your buttocks and thighs back and apart (see pages 87–88). Rest your forearms on the table.
3. Place your feet on the block with your heels lifted up and touching each other. Face the soles of the feet toward each other as much as possible and press them together.

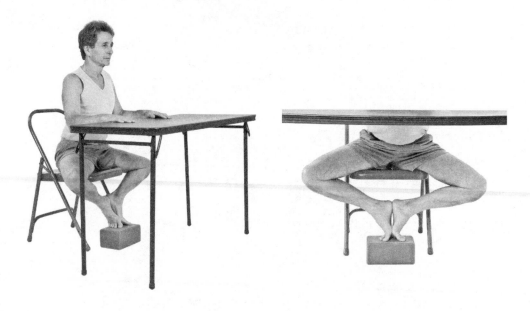

4. Inhale and lift up through your entire spine. Leaning forward slightly, maintain the widening of your sitting bones, then curl your tailbone down. While doing this, stay lifted through your spine. Lean on the table.

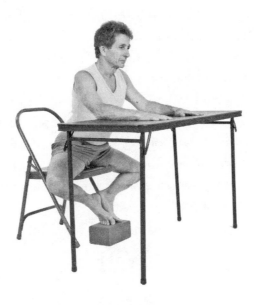

5. Stay centered in your pelvis and spread out from there through all parts of your body. Widen your thighs as much as possible while still pressing your feet together.

6. When you are ready, release the pose and place your feet on the floor.

OSTEOPENIA VARIATION

Props: A yoga mat, two or more blankets, a small towel, and two or four blocks.

1. Fold one or two blankets and stack them on your mat. Place a block on each side.

2. Sit on one corner of the blankets and place the soles of your feet together.

3. Manually adjust your buttocks back and apart (see pages 87–88).

4. If your knees are higher than your hips, add one more blanket under

your hips. If your knees feel strain, you can support them with rolled blankets or additional blocks.

5. Fold the towel and place it under your heels, but not the feet as a whole. This prop will help to align foot, shin, and knee properly.

6. Sit tall and place your hands on the blocks to your sides. Pull your shoulders back and lift up your front chest.

7. Inhale and push down into the blocks to help you raise your lower back. Root down through your pelvic bones.

8. Lift your abdomen in and up as you lengthen the tailbone down. Maintain a slight arch in your lumbar spine as you do this.

9. From the core of your pelvis, simultaneously stretch out through your thighs, down into the blankets, and up through your spine. Expand from the inside out. Your knees will gradually come to the floor as your inner thighs release.

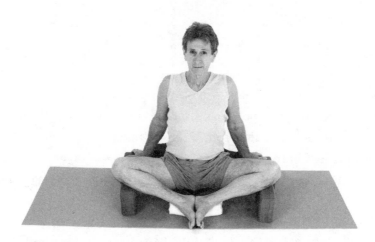

10. Come out of the pose by stretching your legs straight out in front of you, then turning to one side.

PREVENTION VARIATION

Props: A yoga mat, a folded blanket, a chair, and an optional towel.

1. Place a folded blanket on your mat. Sit on a corner of the folded blanket with the soles of your feet together. A towel under your ankles

will relieve knee pain by aligning your feet and shins properly. Set the chair facing you.

2. Manually adjust your buttocks back and apart (see pages 87–88).

3. Sit tall and place your hands on the floor at your sides. Pull your shoulders back and lift up your front chest.

4. Inhale and push down into the floor with your hands to help you raise your lower back. Root down through your pelvic bones.

5. Lift your abdomen in and up as you lengthen the tailbone down. Maintain a slight arch in your lumbar spine as you do this.

6. Press the soles of your feet together while simultaneously stretching your knees to the side.

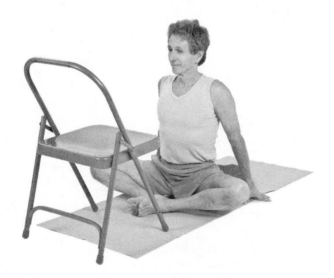

7. As you exhale, bend forward from the hips, with your spine long and your chest still lifted. Lean on the chair seat for support and hold the pose steadily. Rest your head on the chair if that is comfortable. Continue the actions in the legs.

8. From the core of your pelvis, simultaneously stretch out through your thighs, down into the floor through your hips, and up through your spine. Expand from the inside out. Your knees will gradually come down to the floor as your inner thighs release.

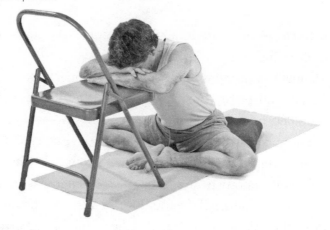

9. Come out of the pose by sitting upright, stretching your legs straight
   out in front of you, then turning to one side.

For a deeper version of this pose, incline forward to put your head on a
block. Lengthen the spine and use the arms actively.

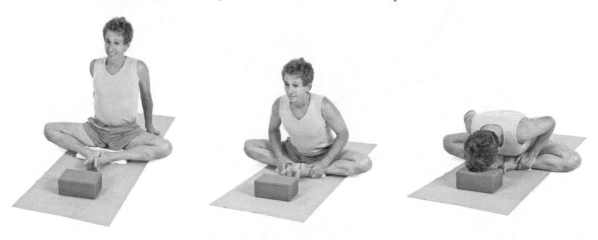

8. BHARADVAJASANA
Twist with Legs to One Side

Purpose: To twist the spine, exerting asymmetrical stress on pelvis and
lumbar and thoracic vertebrae.

Contraindications: Recent herniated lumbar or lower thoracic disc, severe lumbar scoliosis, total hip replacement, ischial bursitis, colostomy, recently fractured rib, pregnancy for all variations.

Props: A chair and a table.

Avoiding pitfalls: Retain the position of the legs as you turn your spine. Avoid twisting by the power of the arms alone; use a spiraling action in the oblique muscles that connect your ribs to your pelvis to twist.

OSTEOPOROSIS VARIATION

1. Place a chair alongside a table, facing to the right.
2. Sit on the chair and bend both of your lower legs to your right, away from the table.
3. Manually widen your buttocks and upper thighs apart (see pages 87–88).
4. Inhaling, expand up through your torso and root down through your pelvic bones into the chair. Attempt to do this evenly on the right and left sides. Firm your leg muscles to hold your legs steady for the twist.

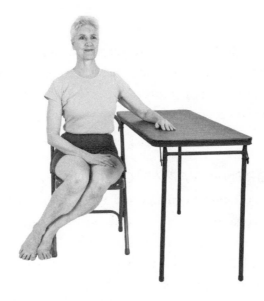

5. As you exhale, twist your torso toward the table, using your stable pelvis as a foundation. Place your hands on the table without raising either shoulder.

6. Firm your abdominal muscles and initiate the twist from your right lower ribs. Twist around the axis of your spine as much as possible.

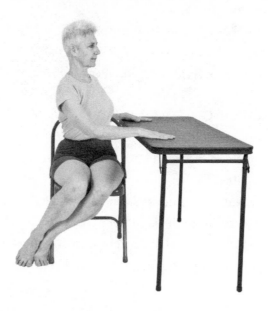

7. Hold the twist for several breaths, stretching up through your spine. Turn from the inside, remaining soft, even as you press down on the table to lift your spine more.
8. Exhale as you revolve back to center.
9. Repeat on the second side.

OSTEOPENIA VARIATION

Contraindications: Pregnancy and all listed for osteoporosis variation.
Props: A yoga mat, a blanket, and two blocks.
Avoiding pitfalls: Retain the position of the legs as you turn your spine.

1. Place a folded blanket on your mat. Sit on the blanket with your legs folded under you, blocks to your left.
2. Move your hips to the left, settling your left hip onto the corner of a block. Your feet are to the right, with the left toes in the arch of the right foot. Both knees are on the floor.
3. Manually pull your buttocks back and apart (see pages 87–88).

4. Inhale and stretch up through your spine. Keep the legs very steady and retract your abdomen.

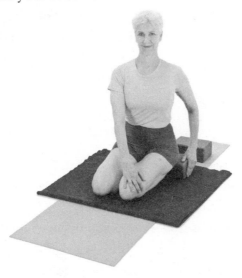

5. Exhale as you turn to your left. Reach your left hand behind you onto the second block, moving it as needed. Place your right hand outside your left knee.
6. Deepen the twist with a wrapping action that begins behind your back right ribs and moves to the left. Turn your ribs and shoulders around the axis of your spine.
7. Stabilize your pelvis and legs by pulling your right leg back into the pelvis. This will give more leverage to the twist of your spine.

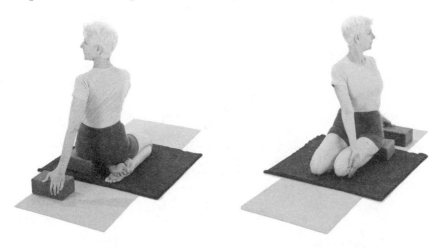

8. Continue to enhance the pose as you breathe: inhale and lift the spine, exhale and turn farther.

9. Level your shoulders; maintain a quiet face as you turn. Soften your diaphragm while maintaining strength in the arms and legs. Move farther with each exhalation.

10. Inhale as you return to center.

11. Repeat on the second side.

PREVENTION VARIATION

Props: A yoga mat and two blankets.

Contraindications: Pregnancy and all listed for osteoporosis variation.

Avoiding pitfalls: Use enough support under your hips to orient your pelvis vertically (without tipping back) and place both knees on the floor. Do not twist by the power of the arms alone; use the oblique muscles that connect your ribs to your pelvis to twist.

1. Place a folded blanket on your mat. Sit on the blanket with your legs folded under you and a folded blanket to your left.

2. Move your hips to the left, settling your left hip onto the corner of the blanket. Your feet are to the right, with the left toes in the arch of the right foot, as in the osteopenia variation (see pages 262–64).

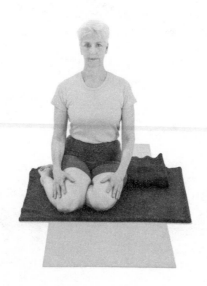

3. Manually pull your buttocks back and apart (see pages 87–88).

4. Inhale and stretch up through your spine. Keep the legs very steady and retract your abdomen.

5. Exhale as you turn to your left. Reach your left hand behind you on the floor; place your right hand on your left knee.

6. Deepen the twist with a wrapping action that begins behind your right back ribs and moves to the left. Turn your ribs and shoulders around the axis of your spine.

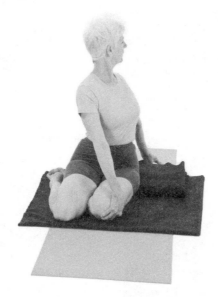

7. Stabilize your pelvis and legs by pulling your right leg back into the pelvis. This will give more leverage to the twist of your spine.

8. Continue to enhance the pose as you breathe: inhale and lift the spine, exhale and turn more.

9. Level your shoulders; maintain a quiet face as you turn. Soften your diaphragm while maintaining strength in the arms and legs. Move farther with each exhalation.

10. Inhale as you return to center.

11. Repeat on the second side.

These pictures illustrate how to get into the full pose with one leg in Lotus Pose and one arm wrapped behind to catch the toes. Practice this pose only if you can practice Lotus Pose without knee pain.

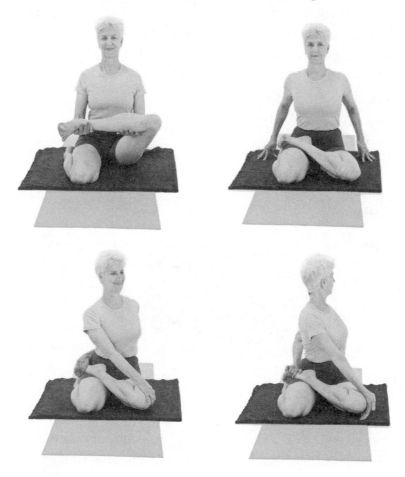

9. SIRSASANA   Progressive Stages to Headstand

Special note: These versions of headstand are safe provided that you observe the contraindications and follow the text.

Purpose: Builds strength in upper back and arms, improves balance, strengthens breathing apparatus, increases blood flow to upper lung fields, builds confidence and quiets the mind.

Contraindications: Glaucoma, macular degeneration, cerebrovascular disease, cervical spondylolisthesis or retrolisthesis, herniated cervical disc, vaso-vagal disorder, carotid body and carotid sinus disorders and arrhythmias.

Props for first variation: A yoga mat, a blanket, and a wall.

Avoiding pitfalls: Set your arm and hand position carefully. In the inverted variations, reach up strongly with your pelvis as you go into the pose.

OSTEOPOROSIS VARIATION

Note: No weight is borne on the head in this preparation pose.

1. Kneel on your mat, using a blanket to pad your knees. Interlace your fingers together, but leave about four inches between your wrists and

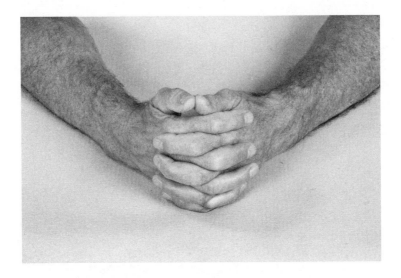

some space between your palms. Your hands will curve very slightly inward toward the midline.

2. With your elbows shoulder-width apart, place your forearms on the mat, positioning your hands carefully. The wrist creases are perpendicular to the floor, thumbs directly over the little finger side of the wrists.

3. Walk your knees back a few inches to allow some stretch in your shoulders and sides. Your shoulder blades are important supports in this pose; retract them so they move toward each other and in toward the ribs.

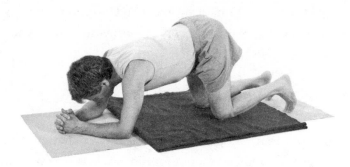

4. Press your forearms down into the floor with steady strength in your arms and shoulders.
5. Firm your abdomen and lift your knees a bit off the floor. Retain a long spine as do this: it will be easier as your knees rise. Do not lose the strength of your arms in the process.

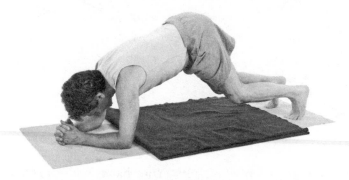

6. Bring your knees down and rest, then repeat several times, lifting your knees and holding the lift for 10 to 20 seconds.
7. Rest in any comfortable position on the floor.

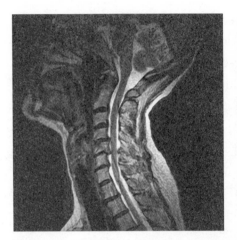
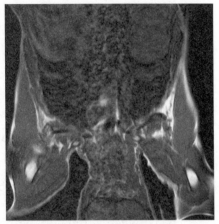

Figure 36. *The left MRI shows why retrolisthesis prohibits headstand. Even when erect, the fifth cervical vertebra threatens the integrity of the spinal cord. In headstand (right), the inverted domes of the muscular diaphragm are weighted down by the abdominal contents, increasing the work of its contraction during inhalation, strengthening all the muscles of respiration, and stimulating the ribs and spine, to which they are attached.*

OSTEOPENIA VARIATION

Note: This variation requires the assistance of a friend or teacher. No weight is borne on the head in this preparation pose.

1. Place your mat perpendicular to a wall. Fold the mat and place a folded blanket between two layers of the mat as shown.

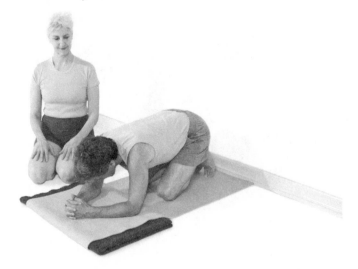

2. Kneel on the floor with your heels a few inches from the wall and interlace the fingers of your hands. Leave a few inches between your wrists and some space between your palms.

3. With your elbows shoulder-width apart, place your lower arms and hands on the mat. You can guess at the distance from the wall according to your height; it should be roughly a leg-length. The thumb sides of your wrists remain directly over the little finger sides.

4. Walk your knees back a few inches to allow some stretch in your shoulders and the sides of your torso. Your shoulder blades are important supports in this pose as they press against the back ribs. Soften the spine between your shoulder blades.

5. Press your forearms down into the mat with steady strength in your arms.

6. Walk your feet up the wall, raising your sitting bones. Do not let your spine curve forward as you do this. The goal is for your pelvis to come directly over your shoulders, inverting your entire upper body. A friend's hand gently pushing your upper back toward the wall while first learning this pose will prevent you from falling backward.

7. Your upper arms stretch to support and lift your shoulders as you raise your pelvis more and more. Your head does not touch the floor.

8. It is not necessary to straighten your legs; the lower body is only helping to invert the upper body.

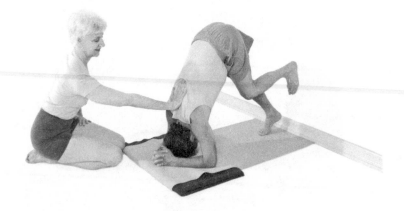

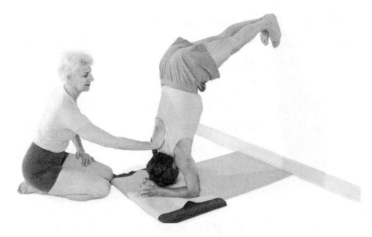

9. Stay up for 10 to 20 seconds or until your arms tire, then walk down carefully and rest in Balasana (see page 210).

PREVENTION VARIATION #1

Note: The body is fully inverted with the support of the wall.

1. Fold your mat into four layers (with an optional blanket inside the layers for padding). Place it on the floor perpendicular to a wall.
2. Come down onto your hands and knees and interlace your fingers. Leave a few inches between your wrists and some space between your palms.
3. Place your lower arms and hands on the mat, your elbows shoulder-width apart and your knuckles about two inches from the wall.

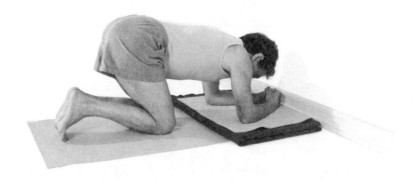

4. Walk your knees back to lengthen your torso.

5. Your shoulder blades still give important support in this pose. With your arms strong, move your upper chest toward the floor somewhat and strongly connect your shoulder blades onto your back, moving them toward each other and in toward your body. Broaden your ribs in front. This is essential for supporting your body properly.

6. Lift your hips up, come onto your toes, and walk in toward the wall. Your head touches the floor lightly.

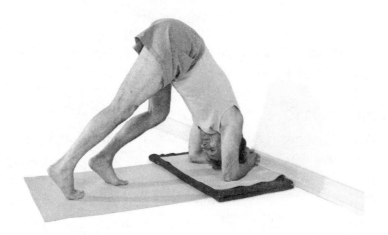

7. Pause to breathe and renew the strength of your shoulders, arms, upper back, and abdomen.

8. Bring one leg in closer to you and reach the other leg back, stretching it straight. Carefully and with control, swing the back leg up, followed by the second leg, bringing both feet to the wall. Kicking up with straight legs will give you more control and power.

9. Now that you are inverted, repeat the actions that support the pose: press down through your wrists and forearms, and lift your shoulder blades up away from the floor enough to lift your head off as well.

10. Flex your feet and stretch all ten toes. Press your legs and ankles together for stability.

11. Actively stretch down through your head and neck and up through your legs and feet.

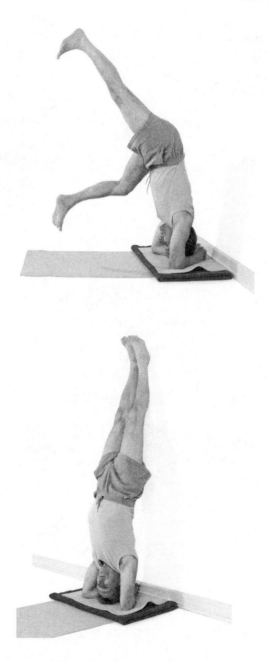

12. Remain in the pose for 20 to 30 seconds at first, gradually increasing the time when ready. To come down, bend your knees, touch your toes down, and rest in Balasana (see page 210).

PREVENTION VARIATION #2

Purpose: With weight on the head, there is compressive stimulation of cervical and thoracic vertebrae. This pose builds strength in the upper back and arms, improves balance, strengthens breathing apparatus, increases blood flow to upper lung fields, and quiets the mind.

1. Follow steps 1–5 from Prevention Variation #1.
6. Place the crown of your head on the mat, with the back of your head touching the base of your thumbs. Lift your hips up, come onto your toes, and walk in toward the wall.

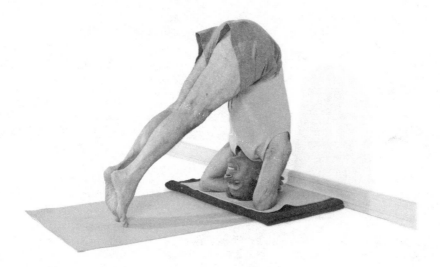

7. Pause to breathe and recharge the strength of your shoulders, arms, upper back, and abdomen.
8. There are several ways to invert the legs. Swing with one straight leg and then the other (easiest and safest way), or hop with both legs bent, or raise both straight legs together (most elegant).
9. Once you are inverted, perform the actions that support the pose: press down through your wrists and forearms and lift your shoulder blades up away from the floor.

10. Flex your feet and stretch all ten toes. Press your legs together for stability.

11. Actively stretch vertically: down through your head and neck and up through your legs and feet.

12. Remain in the pose for up to 5 minutes. To come down, bend your knees, touch your toes down, and rest in Balasana (see page 210).

13. Perform this pose farther away from the wall when you feel secure.

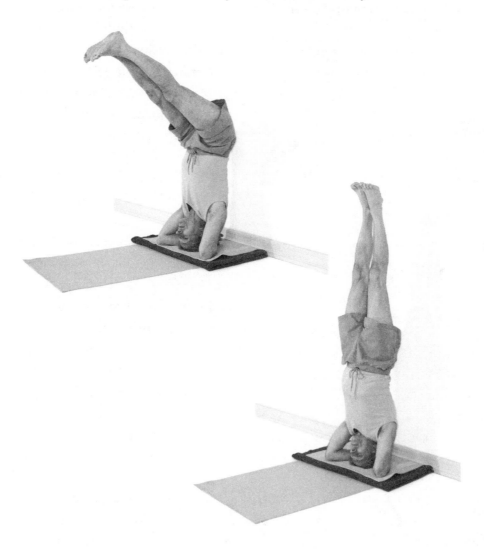

10. SALAMBA SARVANGASANA
Progressive Stages to Shoulder Stand

OSTEOPOROSIS VARIATION #1

Purpose: Stimulates the cervical and thoracic spine, prepares for the full pose.

Contraindications: Herniated cervical disc, severe cervical arthritis.

Props: A belt.

Avoiding pitfalls: Keep your upper back erect but not rigid. Avoid overly tightening your throat. Avoid overarching your lower back.

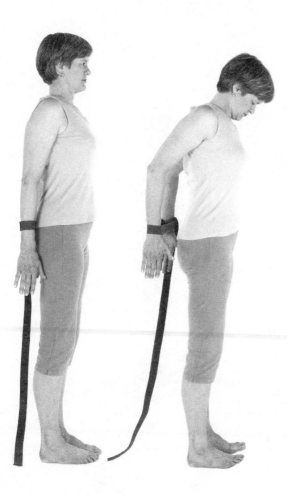

1. Make a 10- to 12-inch loop in a belt. Stand, and with your arms behind you loop the belt around your wrists.
2. Inhale and lift your whole torso, making your sides very long.
3. Retract your shoulder blades to support this tall posture. Pull your upper arms back.
4. Press your arms out to the sides against the belt.
5. Inhale again and lengthen up through your neck.
6. Exhaling, move your head forward and down toward your chest until you feel a good stretch through the back of your neck.
7. Stay for several breaths, then inhale and raise your head.
8. Release your arms from the belt.

OSTEOPOROSIS VARIATION #2

Practicing Ustrasana is a good preparation for Shoulder Stand. Follow all directions for the osteoporosis variation of that pose (see pages 176–78).

OSTEOPENIA VARIATION

Purpose: To stimulate the posterior aspects of all vertebrae, pelvis and leg bones. To prepare for the full pose without inversion or intense stretch in the cervical spine.

Contraindications: Cerebrovascular disease, severe cervical spondylolisthesis.

Props: A yoga mat, two or three blankets, a block, and a chair.

Avoiding pitfalls: Contract all muscles equally from your feet to your shoulders while breathing smoothly. Avoid overarching your lower back: make the body one long line with your abdominal muscles active.

1. Place two or three neatly folded blankets at one end of your mat, a block in the center of the mat, and a chair at the other end facing inward. Stack the blankets with the neatly folded edges lined up and facing away from the other props.

2. Lie on the floor with your shoulders on the folded edge of the blankets, your head on the floor, and your pelvis on the block. Place your upper arms close to your sides and bend your elbows to point the fingers straight up, palms facing in.

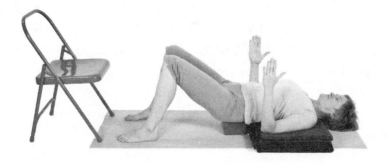

3. Place your heels on the chair seat, adjusting the placement of the chair as needed.

4. Bring your awareness to the full length of your body. The name *Sarvangasana* means "all-limb pose"; prepare to use the entire body to perform this pose.

5. Press your shoulders, upper arms, and feet down strongly and lift the rest of your body away from the props. Maintain steady strength as you breathe calmly. Your shoulder blades retract onto your back, your chest expands and lifts up, and your tailbone lengthens toward the chair.

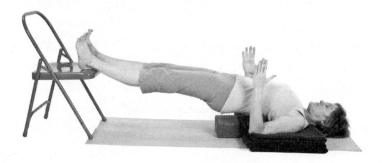

6. Hold the pose for 10 to 30 seconds, then come down and bend your knees.

7. Roll to one side to come off the props.

PREVENTION VARIATION #1

Caution: This variation and the next one should be practiced under the supervision of an experienced teacher. Proper use of props and positioning of the shoulders is crucial. The two Prevention variations of Sarvangasana should not be done by people with osteopenia or osteoporosis—vertebral fractures could occur. These poses are intended as preventive, not curative. The same pressure that might break a weakened vertebral body will stress an intact one and actually strengthen it, preventing the very fractures which later would prohibit the pose!

Purpose: To stimulate the upper arms, thoracic spine, and pelvic bones.

Contraindications: Cerebrovascular disease, glaucoma, macular degeneration, vaso-vagal syndrome.

Props: A chair, two yoga mats, a block, and three blankets.

Avoiding pitfalls: If you find it difficult to tuck your shoulders under you due to stiffness in your thoracic or cervical spine, use another blanket under your shoulders.

1. Place a chair on your mat, a folded mat on the chair seat, and the blankets on the floor in front of the chair. Fold the blankets so that the neatly folded edge faces out from the chair; this edge will support your shoulders.

2. Lie down with your head and neck off the blankets, your shoulders two inches from the folded edge, giving yourself extra space to roll up onto your shoulders. Place your hips on the block.

3. Place your feet or lower legs on the chair seat and grasp the front legs of the chair with your hands. Avoid rounding your back as you do these things.

4. Inhale and expand your chest from the inside.

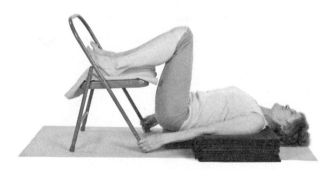

5. With your knees parallel, press down into the chair seat to lift your hips straight up. Reposition your feet flat on the chair seat.

6. One shoulder at a time, tuck your upper arms under you toward your spine so that the tops of your shoulders come onto the blanket. This will take pressure off your neck and allow you to go into the pose

more deeply. Your weight must be borne by the tops of your shoulders, not your neck.

7. With each inhalation, lift your chest and pelvis up more. With each exhalation, lengthen from your chest to your knees. Press down into the blankets with your shoulders to lift more. The more you press down, the more the pose will expand upward.

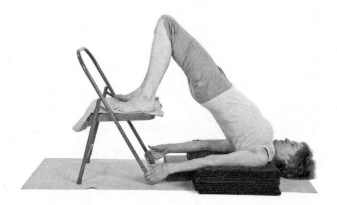

8. To intensify the pose, lift one foot off the chair and stretch the leg up and directly over your head. Stretch strongly through the leg all the way to your heel and toes. Full action in this leg will lighten the pose.

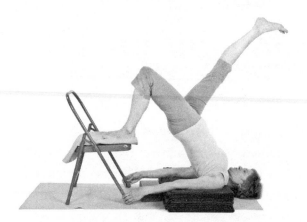

9. After 10 to 20 seconds, return that leg to the chair. Perform the same action with the other leg.

10. To come out of the pose, place the foot on the chair, roll your pelvis back down to the floor, and rest.

PREVENTION VARIATION #2

Purpose: To increase pressure on anterior cervical and thoracic vertebrae and posterior pelvic bones; to increase blood flow to superior lung fields. Support from the wall helps the spine to elongate and allows you to hold the pose for a longer time.

Contraindications: Imbalance, cerebrovascular disease, glaucoma, macular degeneration, vaso-vagal syndromes, herniated cervical disc, severe cervical stenosis from any cause.

Props: A yoga mat, four or five blankets, a block, a wall, and an optional belt.

Avoiding pitfalls: The shoulders and upper arms are your foundation in this pose, so take special care to position them as instructed. Make sure that your shoulders are tucked behind you toward your spine before stretching up into the full inversion. Weight should be borne on the shoulders, not on the neck. If your elbows are wider apart than your shoulders, it is a sign that you may need another blanket under your shoulders to establish a good foundation in the pose. A belt can also secure your upper arms in the correct position.

1. Place your mat perpendicular to a wall. Fold the mat to bring its far edge about 24 inches from the wall (more if you are taller). Fold your blankets so that one edge is neat and firm and the width accommodates your shoulders. Stack three or four of them on the end of the mat, with the firm edge away from the wall. Place the extra fold of the yoga mat over the blankets; this will support your elbows in the pose. Place the block between the wall and the stack of blankets.

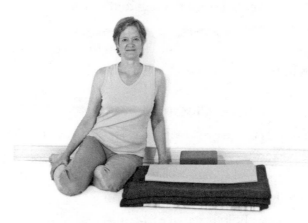

2. Sit with your back to the wall near the blankets.

3. Roll to lie down so that your shoulders are on the neatly folded edge, your head is on the floor, and your hips are on the block close to the wall. Your feet are on the wall, knees bent. Adjust your distance from the wall as needed.

4. Pause to breathe and soften. Shrug your shoulders slightly toward your ears and tuck them under toward your spine.

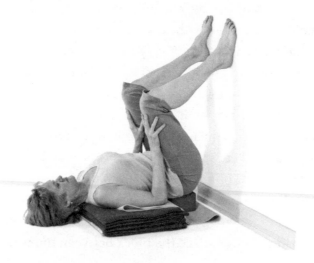

5. Press your feet into the wall and pull your pelvis up. Bring your hands onto your back. Continue to press your shoulders down as your pelvis lifts up more and more.

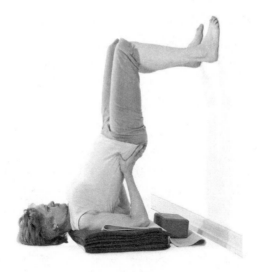

6. Lift your knees and tailbone very strongly to remain vertical over your shoulders.
7. Align your elbows shoulder-width apart. If this is challenging, use a belt loop around your arms just above your elbows. (See Prevention Variation #3, steps 1 and 2.)

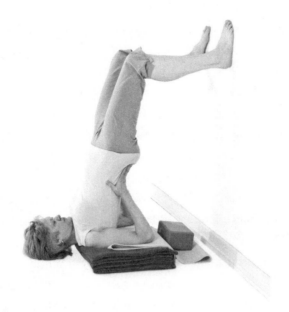

8. If you feel steady and lifted, bring one or both feet away from the wall and stretch them straight up.

9. Remain in the pose for as long as you wish, then roll down softly. Stretch your chest over the edge of the blankets to rest. Then roll to one side to come up.

PREVENTION VARIATION #3

We include the full pose in this section because we consider it to be such an excellent preventive pose. It is essential to practice all the preceding variations first to achieve the necessary strength and familiarity to do this pose safely.

These instructions call for three to five blankets to bring the body's weight over the shoulders rather than the neck. It is crucial to avoid excess flexion pressure on the posterior thoracic and cervical vertebrae, which may lead to injury.

However, a higher stack of blankets introduces a risk of slipping off onto the floor. Our advice is to start with three blankets and to limit the flexion required of the neck. As your balance improves, you may add more blankets to lift higher.

Purpose: Improve balance; increase pressure on anterior cervical and thoracic vertebrae and posterior pelvic bones; increase blood flow to superior lung fields, and stimulate the thyroid and parathyroid glands. This pose is calming to the nervous system, a good way to conclude a practice.

Contraindications: Imbalance, cerebrovascular disease, glaucoma, macular degeneration, vaso-vagal syndromes, herniated cervical disc, severe cervical stenosis, severe hypertension.

Props: A yoga mat, three to five blankets, a block, and an optional belt.

Avoiding pitfalls: The shoulders and upper arms are your foundation in this pose. Although the neck receives a strong stretch, it should not bear much weight. Make sure that your shoulders are tucked behind you toward your spine before stretching up into the full inversion. If your elbows are wider apart than your shoulders, your spine may sag and you may need another blanket under your shoulders to establish a good foundation in the pose. A higher stack of blankets may feel unstable at first, but will help you create the correct foundation on your shoulders, not your neck. A belt can also secure your upper arms in the correct position.

1. Fold three to five blankets so that one edge is neat and firm and the width accommodates your shoulders. Stack them on a yoga mat, and fold the yoga mat over the edge to support your elbows. Place the block at the edge of the blankets and sit on it. Prepare the belt by making a loop the same width as your shoulders. The picture below shows how to measure the belt. Once you have the correct width, take the belt off one arm to proceed with the next instruction.

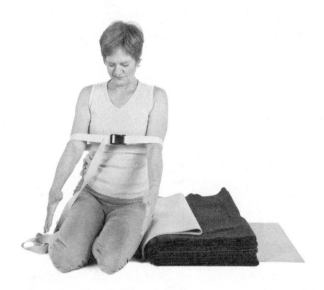

2. Place the belt around your arms from behind, the way you would put on a jacket. Secure the belt just above your elbows, and lie down with your shoulders on the neat folded edge, your head on the floor, and your hips on the block. Bend your knees.

3. Pause to breathe and soften. Shrug your shoulders slightly toward your ears and tuck them under toward your spine.

4. When you are ready to go up, swing your feet and legs overhead. As soon as possible, put your hands on the back of your pelvis.

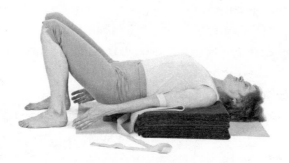

5. Pause again and breathe.

6. Stretch your legs up to bring your pelvis more over your shoulders and your whole body up into the inverted position. As your back ribs lift, adjust your hands lower toward your shoulder blades. Placing your hands in contact with your skin will provide good traction to lift.

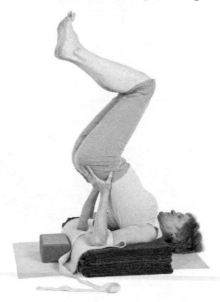

7. Aided by the belt, squeeze your elbows into toward the midline and press your upper arms down to get more lift in the pose.

8. If you feel excess pressure on your head or neck, come down and add more blanket support.

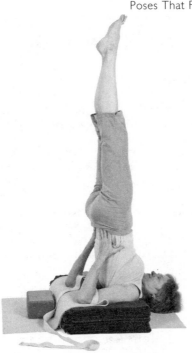

9. Breathe smoothly and relax your face, but maintain strength in your arms and spine as you hold the pose. Stretch your legs up and spread your toes.

10. To come down, roll slowly down to the props. Adjust your position so that your head is on the blankets; move the block to support your pelvis.

11. Rest here. When you are ready, roll to the side to come up.

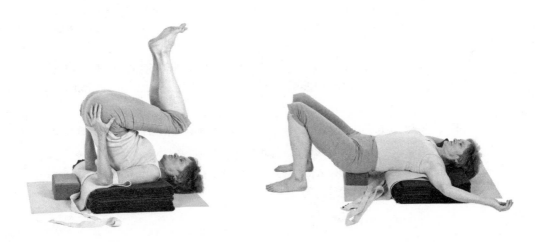

11. SAVASANA   Corpse Pose

Purpose: To cease effort, relax, assimilate, and consolidate gains.

Contraindications: Late pregnancy.

Props: A yoga mat, three blankets, optional eye cover.

Avoiding pitfalls: After the initial setup, avoid fussing and fidgeting, become settled. B. K. S. Iyengar commented in *Light on Yoga*, "By remaining motionless for some time and keeping the mind still while you are fully conscious, you learn to relax. This conscious relaxation invigorates and refreshes both body and mind. But it is much harder to keep the mind than the body still. Therefore, this apparently easy posture is one of the most difficult to master."

1. Make sure the space is quiet and safe from distractions.

2. Fold one blanket to support a slight arch of your thoracic spine, roll the second for under your knees, and fold the third one to support your neck and head. An eye cover may help to relax your face and allow you to retreat from all outer stimuli.

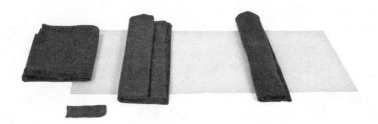

3. Lie on your back with arms at your sides, palms up. Make sure that the chest-supporting blanket allows your shoulders to be flat on the floor. Refold or adjust as necessary.

4. Adjust your hips by turning your legs inward to widen the back of the pelvis, then let the feet roll apart as you relax.

5. Lengthen your buttocks away from the waist if you feel any compression in your lower back.

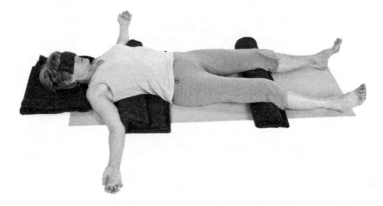

6. Tuck your shoulder blades gently in toward the spine to open the front of your chest.

7. Make sure that your neck is long and your chin and forehead are level. Then guide your attention through your whole body systematically from head to toe and back again, letting each part relax thoroughly.

8. Do not fret if your mind produces thoughts; just watch them unemotionally without being drawn into the content. Be a compassionate witness. You might notice yourself reviewing an event, thinking of a person, or making a plan. Try not to follow the pull of any thoughts, but passively observe them come and go. Trust in the process of letting go.

9. After 5 to 10 minutes of quiet rest, take a few deeper breaths, stretch your arms and legs gently, bend your knees, and softly roll to the side. Take your time getting up, and respect whatever effects, changes, and benefits you may feel from your yoga practice. Remember your intention. Affirm your process of growth and healing.

Afterword

Osteoporosis and osteoarthritis (as well as heart disease, diabetes, and obesity) are chronic conditions that put limits on one's life expectancy, employment opportunities, and quality of life.[1] Medications and hormone replacement therapies are rarely a realistic option for the 200 million sufferers. For that reason, this book supports research in yoga for the prevention and treatment of osteoporosis.

We are encouraged by our observations of those who are reaping the benefits of yoga therapy, and we'd be interested in hearing about your experience. Joining our study is easy: Simply get a DEXA scan around the time you start practicing yoga and send it to us. If your DEXA scan indicates that you have osteopenia or osteoporosis, there are some additional tests we recommend. (If you are anywhere within the normal range, and wish to do yoga for prevention, you do not need the additional tests.) Once we have the DEXA scan and any other results that were necessary, we'll send you a DVD with a 10- to 12-minute program that demonstrates the categories of poses you've seen in this book: Osteoporosis, Osteopenia, and Preventive. Do the poses faithfully and get another DEXA scan after two years. Even though we'd like you to do yoga every day, your data will be useful to us regardless of how rarely or often you do it. The DVD is provided without cost; your only obligation is to yourself.

For more information, go to sciatica.org, where you'll find an induction form, a newsletter, a bulletin board for those in the study, and contact information.

Now that you've read this book, it's time to actually do the yoga! We hope that we have encouraged those readers who are new to yoga to try it out and experience yoga's many blessings. No one is too old to do yoga, and the earlier in life you start, the better it is for your bones. If you already practice yoga, you may find some new poses here which will enhance your practice and provide you with more variety and benefit.

We hope the book will give you ways to *think* about yoga and intelligently assess what you're doing, rather than blindly obeying the words of others. That's not what yoga is about!

Follow the directions mindfully, proceeding with caution but also confidence and courage. Listen to your body's signals. You may feel soreness at first, as the muscles get used to working and stretching. With practice, you can distinguish between the heaviness of lethargy that will dissipate as you move and a different kind of fatigue that tells you to stop and rest. You may be surprised: Many students say that as they begin to practice, the pleasure of moving inspires them to do more than they thought they could. Every effort you make will pay off, strengthening your bones as well as improving your overall health.

Yoga is nontoxic and free, vigorous yet peaceful and relaxing. It is good for your heart, your lungs, your brain, your circulation, your bones and joints, and your muscles. Yoga does nothing to injure the environment. In fact, you, dear reader, are part of the environment. Don't you want to improve the environment?

Alphabetical List of Poses

Poses by Chapter

Chapter Eleven: Poses That Focus on Balance

Glossary

abduction: Movement away from the midline. Lifting one's arms out to the side abducts them.

acromegaly: Swelling of hands, feet, facial features, and internal organs caused by increased secretion of growth hormone by the pituitary gland, often due to pituitary tumor.

acromioclavicular joint: The joint connecting the clavicle with the acromion, a superolateral boney projection of the scapula.

adduction: Movement toward the midline, even crossing it. To touch the left shoulder with the right hand one must adduct the right arm.

ankylosing spondylitis: Progressive inflammation and eventual fusion of vertebral bodies, largely in males; hereditary. Fusion and virtual rigidity of the spine is frequently complete by the early 20s, yielding a stooped or hunched thorax.

architectonic: The arrangement of supporting forces within a structure.

arthritis: Destructive inflammation of a joint or joints. When referring to types of arthritis, the plural is *arthritides,* in the manner of ancient Greek.

atomic force microscopy: Very high resolution probe that measures a local property such as height or magnetic force by placing a micromachined tip close to the sample.

autosomal: Trait or condition that is determined by genes carried and inherited in the nongender portion of the chromosomes. The traits may be dominant (requiring only one gene from one parent) or recessive (requiring the gene from both parents), or may have a more complex relationship to the individual's genetic makeup.

axon: The thin extended outgrowth from a neuron cell body that normally propagates impulses away from that cell body toward another neuron, a muscle, or a gland. It derives from the Greek word for *axis*.

bisphosphonates: Any synthetic analog of pyrophosphate that is used in treating osteoporosis to inhibit the action of osteoclasts, which resorb and thereby weaken bone. Examples include Fosamax, Actonel.

bone quality: Bone's material and structural nature, which determines its strength and resistance to fracture. Its internal and external form as well as its structure. It is often determined in part by atomic force microscopy.

brachial plexus: Region at each side of the neck where nerve roots from the lower cervical spine combine and split again to form the major nerves of the upper extremities such as the median, ulnar, and radial nerves.

bursa: A closed sac with a synovial lining and joint fluid within, generally separating a bone from a tendon. They are thought to evolve from joints, since they have the same basic structure, retained because they usefully prevent the tendon from bruising the bone, and the bone from fraying the tendon. The Latin word *bursa* means "purse."

calcitonin: A hormone secreted by the parafollicular cells of the thyroid that lowers blood calcium. It balances the effects of parathyroid hormone, which raises blood calcium. This relationship regulates calcium metabolism. Synthesized and available under the brand name Miacalcin (salmon calcitonin). An oral preparation is being readied for the U.S. market.

cartilage: The semi-stiff substance that lines joints and forms movable tubes in the body such as the trachea, the nasal cavity, and the Adam's apple. There are three forms: hyaline cartilage, elastic cartilage, and fibrocartilage.

cartilaginous: Made of cartilage.

cauda equina: In adults, the spinal cord proper ends at the lower thoracic or upper lumbar levels above where lumbar nerve roots exit the spinal canal. Collections of nerve fibers descend through the lumbar portion of the canal, giving the appearance of a horse's tail.

Chiari malformations: A range of congenital defects at the base of the skull that may be mild, with dizziness, neuromuscular symptoms, and impaired coordination (Type I); involve defects of the cervical vertebrae and spinal canal that may lead to paralysis (Type II, Arnold-Chiari); or be even more serious, causing hydrocephalus and similar difficulties (Type III).

chondrocytes: Cells that secrete the fibers that constitute cartilage.

collagen: A triple helix of three long protein chains that wrap around one another. Cross-linked molecules of collagen become undistensible (they cannot be stretched) and are stronger than many metals.

collagenase: An enzyme that breaks down collagen into its constituent amino acids.

contralateral: The opposite side. The right is contralateral to the left.

conus medullaris: The enlargement of the spinal cord in the lower thoracic spine where it gives off the fibers for all 5 levels of the lumbar spine below the level at which the cord proper terminates.

cytokine: A protein or glycoprotein between 8 and 30 daltons in size that, like hormones, signals cells and calls forth a number of specific activities at the cellular level.

dendrite: The branching outgrowth from a neuron that acquires impulses that are then transmitted through the cell body to the axon, and hence to another cell. The Greek word for *dendrites* means "pertaining to a tree."

DEXA-scan: Dual energy X-ray absorptiometry, the very low-dose standard examination to determine bone density.

distal: Farther from the point of reference or axis.

eccentric contraction: Muscular effort that resists and controls its relaxation against resistance—for example, how the quadriceps lengthen when you gradually bend your knees.

elastin: Polypeptide (protein) chains that cross-link like collagen, but with the opposite effect: They coil into a form that may uncoil when the fiber is stretched and retract when the stretch is terminated.

estrogen: A female hormone synthesized in the ovaries.

extension: Motion of bones at a joint away from each other, or away from the torso. Exception: Ankle and toe extension brings the foot and toes upward.

external rotation: Clockwise revolving motion of the right arm and leg; counterclockwise revolving motion of the left limbs. At the ankle and wrist, these movements are termed *supination*.

extrude: To send forth, in this context, out of a cell through its membrane.

firm: Used as a verb; to contract a muscle without moving the bones to which it is attached.

flexion: Motion of bones at a joint toward each other, or in closer to the torso. Exception: Ankle and toe flexion points the toes away from the torso.

gait cycle: The repetitive series of movements that each foot, ankle, knee, and hip and the trunk and arms go through with each pair of steps.

glycoprotein: A molecule made up of a carbohydrate and a protein. They are prominent in joint fluid and vital for many immune system functions.

gout: Generally intermittent, extremely painful condition deriving from the body's overproduction of uric acid, a derivative of the nucleic acid purine. It is associated with a protein-rich diet and is related to obesity.

greater trochanter: An outward projection of bone on the proximal femur to which abductors and external rotators of the hip are attached.

growth hormone: A protein substance secreted by the pituitary gland that acts on the liver and other tissues to regulate growth and metabolism. Also known as *somatotropin.*

hydroxyapatite: The mineral and protein amalgam salt that is the major component of bone.

internal rotation: Counterclockwise revolving motion of the right arm and leg; clockwise revolving of the left limbs. At the ankle and wrist, these movements are termed *pronation.*

isometric: Action of contracting a muscle or muscle group without it moving, generally against resistance either from antagonistic muscle or muscle group, or outside force equal to it. In pressing the palms together, one isometrically contracts the pectoralis muscles.

mechanoreception: The capacity of cells to respond to mechanical stimulation, be it in the form of pressure or movement of the cell's membrane, or collision of molecules (for example, hearing, feeling, smell, and taste), or other physical modalities (sight).

metamorphoses: The changing of living organisms from one form to another, as a caterpillar becoming a butterfly.

micro-MRI: A magnetic imaging device that can focus on very small regions and is valuable for determining the structure of bone interior and thus a determinant of bone quality.

multiple myeloma: A malignancy of plasma cells, which produce antibodies. Multiple myeloma has no cure, but is treated with chemotherapy, steroids, and thalidomide. Stem cell transplantation appears to be an effective fourth treatment modality.

myotatic reflex: Contraction of a muscle in response to a sudden stretching force, due to stretch of the intrafusal fibers. Examples include the patellar reflex, the Achilles tendon reflex.

neuroforamen: Anatomical openings between each two vertebrae through which nerve roots pass.

neutral: The position of limbs or torso that is without flexion, extension, abduction, adduction, or external or internal rotation. The entire body in neutral is also known as the *anatomical position*. This is different from the yogi's Savasana, in which arms and legs are somewhat externally rotated.

nonsteroidal anti-inflammatory: Medications related to aspirin that interfere with prostaglandin-mediated pathways that generate pain and enhance inflammation. These medicines reduce both pain and inflammatory responses such as swelling and redness. However, they have varying degrees of side effects associated with their use, such as gastric irritation, ulcer, and prolonged bleeding time. Examples are Motrin, Relafen, Voltaren, Celebrex, and Mobic.

normal distribution: A totally random array of values; standard deviations indicate the probability of a given value, for example, 1 in 10 or 1 in 250.

osteitis fibrosis cystica: Fibrous replacement of healthy bone as osteoclasts absorb it. Also known as Recklinghausen's disease of bone, it is caused by an excess of parathyroid hormone, among other conditions that increase the reabsorption of calcium and phosphorus.

osteoarthritis: Erosion of the cartilage at joints, either without single cause or due to trauma. It is characterized by irregular boney outgrowths at the joint and painful restrictions of movement and swelling, mainly of weight-bearing and very active joints. Since chronic conditions are cumulative, it is more common in older persons.

osteoarthropathy: Any disorder that affects bones and joints. Its origins are Greek: *osteo,* bone; *arthron,* joint; *pathos,* suffering.

osteoblast: Cells that lie just outside of bones and are destined to make the protein matrix of the bones.

osteoclast: Large cells containing up to 50 nuclei. They attach to bones and secrete cytokines, which dissolve bones' substance, returning the minerals and proteins to the bloodstream.

osteocyte: Cells descended from osteoblasts, located within the bones, actively secreting the protein matrix that comes to surround them.

osteoid: Protein matrix secreted by osteocytes that attracts calcium, phosphate, and other minerals. Together, these minerals fuse into hydroxyapatite, the basic constituent of bone.

osteomalacia: Insufficient calcification of bones, often due to low vitamin D or kidney dysfunction, in which the bones' osteoid component bends painfully under stresses. It may begin during pregnancy.

osteonecrosis: Death and degeneration of bone tissue within a living individual. A relatively rare occurrence associated with long-term bisphosphonate use and dental procedures.

osteopenia: Low bone mineral density in which the T-score is between −1.0 and −2.5.

osteopetrosis: Excessive trabecular growth and calcification, particularly of long bones, that obliterates the marrow cavities, leading to anemia of varying severity, possibly leading to deafness, blindness, and death. More severe forms are autosomal dominant.

osteophyte: A nonanatomical outgrowth of bone, generally occurring at the joints, where it may limit range of motion and narrow neuroforamina.

parathyroid hormone (PTH): A hormone produced by the parathyroid glands that raises blood calcium levels by simultaneously stimulating bone resorption, reducing calcium excretion by the kidneys, and increasing intestinal absorption. Its effects are modified by calcitonin and other hormones. Synthesized and available under the brand name Forteo.

paraesthesias : Strange sensations such as tingling, pins and needles, insects crawling on the skin. Numbness is when you do not feel what is there; paraesthesias are when you feel what is not there.

perichondrium: Cells lining cartilage, except at joint interfaces; supplies oxygen and nourishes the chondrocytes, the cells that make cartilage.

plantar fasciitis: Painful inflammation of the insertion of the plantar fascia into the calcaneus, also known as *heel spur.*

progesterone: A gender-active steroid hormone that opposes estrogen's effects on the uterus and also helps create and maintain bone. Influencing osteoblasts to become osteocytes, it has been found to increase bone mineral density as much as 10 percent in one year.

proteoglycan: A large molecule found in most vertebrates' bone and cartilage, composed of proteins and glycosaminoglycans (i.e., polysaccharides) such as derivatives of glucosamine and galactosamine.

protraction: Movement of the scapulae or shoulder blades forward, toward the ventral or navel-bearing side of the body. In human anatomy, it is nearly equivalent to abducting them (bringing them away from the spine).

proximal: Closer to the point of reference or axis.

pseudogout: Gout-like episodes caused by calcium pyrophosphate crystals, rather than the urate crystals that irritate the synovial membrane in true gout. It is also associated with calcification of the articular cartilage.

radiculopathy: Compression of or injury to the nerve roots that exit the spine.

resorption: Reabsorption of a substance into the circulatory system.

retraction: Movement of the scapulae or shoulder blades backward, toward the dorsal aspect of the thorax. In human anatomy, it is nearly equivalent to adducting them (bringing them toward the spine).

rheumatoid arthritis: Arthritic damage to the joints resulting from the immune system's actions, generally on the joint capsules' lining or synovium, also eroding the cartilage and the bone itself.

rickets: A condition caused by vitamin D deficiency producing undercalcified bones and subsequent skeletal and growth disturbances, fractures, spasm, weakness, and irritability.

sacroiliac joint: A bilateral synovial joint between the outer edges of the sacrum and the inner edges of the iliac bones.

scapulothoracic: The relationship between the shoulder blade or scapula and the backs of ribs 2–6, a large area over which the shoulder blade normally moves. It is often referred to as a joint, although its size and structure are quite different from any other joint.

sentinel event: An occurrence of greater significance than its immediate medical consequences. A harbinger of change.

sesamoid bone: A bone encapsulated within a tendon. There is one in the flexor tendon of the big toe as it rounds the joint that connects the toe to the foot. The patella is the largest sesamoid bone in the human body.

sigma: See *standard deviation*.

spicules: The small pieces of protein extruded by osteocytes that make up osteoid, the initial ground substance of bone that attracts calcium and phosphorus to become true bone.

spondyloarthropathy: See *ankylosing spondylitis*.

spondylolisthesis: The sliding of one vertebra (generally forward) on the one below it, resulting in narrowing of the central canal, stenosis, or narrowing the neuroforamina. In either case it may cause radiculopathy.

standard deviation: The interval one must consider to include 34.1 percent of the values above or below the mean in a normal distribution. Denoted by the Greek letter sigma σ.

steroid: Biological molecules, including gender hormones and cortisone, containing a five-carbon ring and three rings each of six carbon atoms.

surgical neck: The part of the proximal femur that connects the ball of the hip joint to the shaft.

synapse: The point at which impulses are passed from one neuron to another, generally by neurotransmitter molecules, but sometimes by direct (electrotonic) propagation of the signal. (For more on this, see B. Gutkin and G. B. Ermentrout, "Spikes too kinky in the cortex?" *Nature* 20 [April 2006]: 999–1000.)

synovial fluid: The yellowish-white fluid that bathes each joint. It serves three essential purposes: It is a first-class lubricant; it brings oxygen, food, and protein building blocks to the cartilage of the joint; and it protects the joint from mechanical and biological causes of disruption

synovial membrane: Similar to a gasket; seals the synovial fluid in the joint. It is quite vascular and richly invested with nerves. It secretes and resorbs the synovial fluid and is exquisitely sensitive, causing pain with distension, inflammation, or disruption.

testosterone: A male steroid hormone produced in the testes, but also by ovaries and adrenal cortices. A potent stimulator of bone formation.

Wolff's law: The architectonic of bone follows the lines of force to which that bone is subjected. First formulated by the German surgeon and anatomist Julius Wolff in 1861.

Notes

Authors' Note

1. I. Weinans and P. J. Prendergast, "Adaptation as a dynamical process far from equilibrium," *Bone* 19, no. 2 (August 1996): 143–149.

Introduction

1. M. S. Garfinkel, H. R. Schumacher Jr., et al., "Evaluation of a yoga-based regimen for treatment of osteoarthritis of the hands," *Journal of Rheumatology* 21, no. 12 (December 1994): 2341. I. Haslock, R. Monro, et al., "Measuring the effects of yoga in rheumatoid arthritis," *British Journal of Rheumatology* 33, no. 8 (August 1994): 787–788. S. L. Kolasinski, A. G. Tsai, et al., "Iyengar yoga for treating symptoms of osteoarthritis of the knees: A pilot study," *Journal of Alternative and Complementary Medicine* 11, no. 4 (August 2005): 689–693.

Chapter I

1. National Osteoporosis Foundation (NOF), "Fast facts on osteoporosis," www.nof.org/osteoporosis/diseasefacts.htm (accessed July 2006).
2. C. Cooper, "The crippling consequences of fractures and their impact on quality of life," *American Journal of Medicine* 103 (1997): 12S–17S, discussion 17S–19S.

3. M. M. Iqbal, "Osteoporosis: Epidemiology, diagnosis and treatment," *Southern Medical Journal* 93, no. 1 (2000): 2–18.

4. D. Brixner, "Assessment of the prevalence and costs of osteoporosis treatment options in a real-world setting," *American Journal of Managed Care* 12 (2006): S191–S198.

5. H. W. Minne, W. Pollähne, et al., "Weeks of pain, vertebral body fractures during sleep, invalidism: Save your osteoporosis patients from this fate," *MMW Fortschritte der Medizin* 144, no. 44 (2002): 41–44.

6. S. Khosla and L. J. Melton III, "Osteopenia," *New England Journal of Medicine* 356, no. 22 (2007): 2293–3000.

7. D. M. Kado, T. Duong, et al., "Incident vertebral fractures and mortality in older women: A prospective study," *Osteoporosis International* 14, no. 7 (2003): 589–594.

8. N. E. Lane, "Epidemiology, etiology and diagnosis of osteoporosis," *American Journal of Obstetrics and Gynecology* 194, no. 2 (February 2006): S3–S11.

9. Minne, Pollähne, et al., "Weeks of pain, vertebral body fractures during sleep, invalidism."

10. Ibid.

11. Lane, "Epidemiology, etiology and diagnosis of osteoporosis."

12. Kado, Duong, et al., "Incident vertebral fractures and mortality in older women."

13. Cooper, "The crippling consequences of fractures and their impact on quality of life."

14. Kado, Duong, et al., "Incident vertebral fractures and mortality in older women."

15. S. L. Silverman, M. E. Minshall, et al., "The relationship of health-related quality of life to prevalent and incident vertebral fractures in postmenopausal women with osteoporosis: Results from the multiple outcomes of raloxifene evaluation study," *Arthritis and Rheumatism* 44, no. 11 (2001): 2611–2619.

16. C. H. Whitehead, R. Wundke, and M. Crotty, "Attitudes to falls and injury prevention: What are the barriers to implementing falls prevention strategies?" *Clinical Rehabilitation* 20, no. 6 (June 2006): 536–542. Lane, "Epidemiology, etiology and diagnosis of osteoporosis."

17. S. Boufous, C. Finch, et al., "The epidemiology of hospitalised wrist fractures in older people, New South Wales, Australia," *Bone* 39, no. 5 (November 2006): 1144–1148.

18. Whitehead, Wundke, and Crotty, "Attitudes to falls and injury prevention."

19. J. M. Morse, R. M. Morse, and S. J. Tylko, "Development of a scale to identify the fall-prone patient," *Canadian Journal on Aging* 8, no. 4 (1989): 366–367.

20. L. W. Mui, L. B. Haramati, et al., "Evaluation of vertebral fractures on lateral chest radiographs of inner-city postmenopausal women," *Calcified Tissue International* 73, no. 6 (2003): 550–554.

21. C. I. Rohr, J. M. Clements, and A. Sarkar, "Treatment and prevention practices in postmenopausal women after bone mineral density screening at a community-based osteoporosis project," *Journal of the American Osteopathic Association* 106, no. 7 (July 2006): 396–401.

22. Whitehead, Wundke, and Crotty, "Attitudes to falls and injury prevention."

23. NOF, "Fast facts on osteoporosis," www.nof.org/osteoporosis/diseasefacts .htm.

24. O. Johnell, A. Kanis, et al., "Predictive value of BMD for hip and other fractures," *Journal of Bone and Mineral Research* 20, no. 7 (July 2005): 1185–1194.

25. E. Barrett-Connor, E. S. Siris, et al., "Osteoporosis and fracture risk in women of different ethnic groups," *Journal of Bone and Mineral Research* 20, no. 2 (February 2005): 185–194.

26. S. R. Cummings, D. Bates, and D. M. Black, "Clinical use of bone densitometry: Scientific review," *JAMA* 288, no. 15 (October 2002): 1889–1897.

27. Ibid.

28. D. W. Bates, D. M. Black, and S. R. Cummings. "Clinical use of bone densitometry: Clinical applications." *JAMA* 288, no. 15 (October 2002): 1898–1900.

29. S. Nayak, I. Olkin, et al., " Meta-analysis: Accuracy of quantitative ultrasound for identifying patients with osteoporosis." *Annals of Internal Medicine* 144, no. 11 (June 2006): 832–881.

30. Johnell, Kanis, et al., "Predictive value of BMD for hip and other fractures."

31. Morse, Morse, and Tylko, "Development of a scale to identify the fall-prone patient." I. Razmus, D. Wilson, et al., "Falls in hospitalized children," *Pediatric Nursing* 32, no. 6 (November–December 2006): 568–572.

32. L. A. Ahmed, H. Schirmer, et al., "Validation of the Cummings' risk score; How well does it identify women with high risk of hip fracture: The Tromso study," *European Journal of Epidemiology* 21, no. 11 (2006): 815–822.

Chapter 2

1. G. H. Bell, O. Dunbar, et al., "Variations in strength of vertebrae with age and their relation to osteoporosis. *Calcified Tissue Research* 1 (1967): 75–86. S. K. Eswaran, A. Gupta, et al., "Cortical and trabecular load sharing in the

human vertebral body," *Journal of Bone and Mineral Research* 22 (January 2007): 149–157.

2. D. W. Nicholson, *Finite Element Analysis: Thermomechanics of Solids* (Boca Raton, FL: CRC Press, 2003), 180–181.

3. Silverman, Minshall, et al., "The relationship of health-related quality of life to prevalent and incident vertebral fractures in postmenopausal women with osteoporosis." W. M. Drake et al., "An investigation of the predictors of bone mineral density and response to therapy with alendronate in osteoporotic men," *Journal of Clinical Endocrinology and Metabolism* 88, no. 12 (December 2003): 5759–5765. Lane, "Epidemiology, etiology and diagnosis of osteoporosis."

4. B. R. Gomberg, P. K. Saha, and F. W. Wehrli, "Method for cortical bone structural analysis from magnetic resonance images," *Academic Radiology* 12 (2005): 1320–1332. F. W. Wehrli, "Structural and functional assessment of trabecular and cortical bone by micro magnetic resonance imaging," *Journal of Magnetic Resonance Imaging* 25, no. 2 (February 2007): 390–409. C. L. Benhamou, S. Poupon, et al., "Fractal analysis of radiographic trabecular bone texture and bone mineral density: Two complementary parameters related to osteoporotic fractures," *Journal of Bone and Mineral Research* 16, no. 4 (2001): 697–704. C. H. Chesnut III, S. Majumdar, et al., "Effects of salmon calcitonin on trabecular microarchitecture as determined by magnetic resonance imaging: Results from the QUEST study," *Journal of Bone and Mineral Research* 20, no. 9 (2005): 1548–1561.

5. Z. Magyar and T. Fel, "Treatment of menopausal symptoms—review of the current literature," *Orvosi Hetilap* 147, no. 19 (May 2006): 879–885.

6. R. M. Neer, C. D. Arnaud, et al., "Effect of parathyroid hormone (1-34) on fractures and bone mineral density in postmenopausal women with osteoporosis," *New England Journal of Medicine* 344, no. 19 (2001): 1434–1441.

7. T. Hassenkam, H. L. Jørgensen, and J. B. Lauritzen, "Mapping the imprint of bone by atomic force microscopy," *Anatomical Record, Part A: Discoveries in Molecular, Cellular, and Evolutionary Biology* 288, no. 10 (October 2006): 1087–1094.

Chapter 3

1. E. S. Siris, S. K. Brenneman, et al., "Predictive value of low BMD for 1-year fracture outcomes is similar for postmenopausal women ages 50–64 and 65 and older: Results from the National Osteoporosis Risk Assessment," *Journal of Bone and Mineral Research* 19, no. 8 (2004): 1215–1220. Medscape Medical News,

search results for "osteoporosis," http://search.medscape.com/medscape-search?queryText=osteoporosis (accessed June 6, 2006).

2. Ibid.

3. M. Y. Ng, P. C. Sham, et al., "Effect of environmental factors and gender on the heritability of bone mineral density and bone size," *Annals of Human Genetics* 70, part 4 (July 2006): 428–438.

4. G. Gong, G. Haynatzki, et al., "Bone mineral density of recent African immigrants in the United States," *Journal of the National Medical Association* 98, no. 5 (May 2006): 746–752.

5. D. Seidlová-Wuttke, K. M. Stürmer, et al., "Contrasting effects of estradiol, testosterone and of a black cohosh extract on density, mechanical properties and expression of several genes in the metaphysis of the tibia and on fat tissue of orchidectomized rats," *Maturitas* 55 (August 2006): S64–S74.

6. G. Zaman, H. L. Jessop, et al., "Osteocytes use estrogen receptor alpha to respond to strain but their ERalpha content is regulated by estrogen," *Journal of Bone and Mineral Research* 21, no. 8 (August 2006): 1297–1306.

7. T. Pomerants, V. Tillmann, et al., "The influence of serum ghrelin, IGF axis and testosterone on bone mineral density in boys at different stages of sexual maturity," *Journal of Bone and Mineral Metabolism* 25, no. 3 (2007): 193–197.

8. Ibid.

9. H. H. Malluche, N. Koszewski, et al., "Influence of the parathyroid glands on bone metabolism," *European Journal of Clinical Investigation* 36, suppl. 2 (August 2006): 23–33.

10. Ibid.

11. Neer, Arnaud, et al., "Effect of parathyroid hormone (1-34) on fractures and bone mineral density in postmenopausal women with osteoporosis."

12. L. Barclay and D. Lie, "Exercise program improves osteoporosis," Medscape Medical News, May 25, 2004, http://cme.medscape.com/viewarticle/478726 (accessed July 31, 2008).

13. R. D. Jackson, A. Z. LaCroix, et al., "Calcium plus vitamin D supplementation and the risk of fractures," *New England Journal of Medicine* 354, no. 7 (February 2006): 669–683.

14. M. J. Bolland, P. A. Barber, et al., "Vascular events in healthy older women receiving calcium supplementation: Randomised controlled trial," *BMJ* 336 (February 2008): 262–266; available at www.bmj.com/.

15. J. Hsia, G. Heiss, et al., "Calcium/vitamin D supplements and cardiovascular events," *Circulation* 115 (2007): 846–854. E. D. Michos and R. S. Blumenthal,

"Vitamin D supplementation and cardiovascular disease risk," *Circulation* 115 (2007): 827–828.

16. M. Norval, A. P. Cullen, et al., "The effects on human health from stratospheric ozone depletion and its interactions with climate change," *Photochemical and Photobiological Sciences* 6, no. 3 (March 2007): 232–251.

17. L. Y. Matsuoka, L. Ide, et al., "Sunscreens suppress cutaneous vitamin D3 synthesis," *Journal of Clinical Endocrinology and Metabolism* 64, no. 6 (June 1987): 1165–1168.

18. F. Bandeira, L. Griz, et al., "Vitamin D deficiency: A global perspective," *Arquivos Brasileiros de Endocrinologia and Metabologia* 50, no. 4 (August 2006): 640–646.

19. J. Bakos and P. Mikó, "Vitamin D forming effectiveness of ultraviolet radiation from sunlight in different months in Budapest, Hungary," *Orvosi Hetilap* 148, no. 7 (February 2007): 319–320.

20. A. Akesson, P. Bjellerup, et al., "Cadmium-induced effects on bone in a population-based study of women," *Environmental Health Perspectives* 114, no. 6 (June 2006): 830–834.

21. M. R. Alam, S. M. Kim, et al., "Effects of safflower seed oil in osteoporosis induced-ovariectomized rats," *American Journal of Chinese Medicine* 34, no. 4 (2006): 601–612.

22. M. Franklin, S. Y. Bu, et al., "Dried plum prevents bone loss in a male osteoporosis model via IGF and the RANK pathway," *Bone* 39, no. 6 (August 2006): 1331–1342.

23. O. Barbier, G. Jacquillet, et al., "Acute study of interaction among cadmium, calcium, and zinc transport along the rat nephron in vivo," *American Journal of Physiology: Renal Physiology* 287, no. 5 (November 2004): 1067–1075.

24. George Kessler, *The Bone Density Program* (New York: Ballantine Books, 2000), 75.

25. Ibid.

Chapter 4

1. M. C. Hochbert, D. E. Thompson, et al., "Effect of alendronate on the age-specific incidence of symptomatic osteoporotic fractures," *Journal of Bone and Mineral Research* 20, no. 6 (2005): 971–976.

2. Drake et al., "An investigation of the predictors of bone mineral density and response to therapy with alendronate in osteoporotic men."

3. R. Bartl, S. Götte, et al., "Adherence with daily and weekly administration

of oral bisphosphonates for osteoporosis treatment," *Deutsche Medizinische Wochenschrift* 131, no. 22 (June 2006): 1257–1262. K. J. Loud and C. M. Gordon, "Adolescent Bone Health," *Archives of Pediatrics and Adolescent Medicine* 160, no. 10 (October 2006).

4. Bartl, Götte, et al., "Adherence with daily and weekly administration of oral bisphosphonates for osteoporosis treatment."

5. C. Roux, E. Seeman, et al., "Efficacy of risedronate on clinical vertebral fractures within six months," *Current Medical Research and Opinion* 20, no. 4 (2004): 433–439.

6. D. M. Reid, J.-P. Devogelaer, et al., "A single infusion of zoledronic acid 5 mg is significantly more effective than daily oral risedronate 5 mg in increasing bone mineral density of the lumbar spine, hip, femoral neck and trochanter in patients with glucocorticoid-induced osteoporosis," presented at the European Congress on Clinical and Economic Aspects of Osteoporosis and Osteoarthritis in Istanbul, Turkey, April 11, 2008. S. Silverman et al., "Effectiveness of bisphosphonates on nonvertebral and hip fractures in the first year of therapy: The risedronate and alendronate (REAL) cohort study," *Osteoporosis International* 18, no. 1 (January 2007): 25–34. J. T. Harrington, L. G. Ste-Marie, et al., "Risedronate rapidly reduces the risk for non-vertebral fractures in women with postmenopausal osteoporosis," *Calcified Tissue International* 74 (2004): 129–135.

7. Hoffmann–La Roche Inc., data on file (ref. #161-014), Nutley, NJ. N. B. Watts, P. Geusens, et al., "Relationship between changes in BMD and nonvertebral fracture incidence associated with risedronate: Reduction in risk of nonvertebral fracture is not related to change in BMD," *Journal of Bone and Mineral Research* 20 (2005): 2097–2104. J. H. Ware, "The limitations of risk factors as prognostic tools," *New England Journal of Medicine* 355, no. 25 (December 2006): 2615–2617.

8. M. R. McClung, E. M. Lewiecki, et al., "Denosumab in postmenopausal women with low bone mineral density," *New England Journal of Medicine* 354, no. 8 (February 2006): 821–831. T. J. Beck, E. M. Lewiecki, et al., "Effects of denosumab on the geometry of the proximal femur in postmenopausal women in comparison with alendronate," *Journal of Clinical Densitometry* 11, no. 3 (July–September 2008): 351–359.

9. H. H. Malluche, N. Koszewski, et al., "Influence of the parathyroid glands on bone metabolism," *European Journal of Clinical Investigation* 36, suppl. 2 (August 2006): 23–33.

10. M. A. McTiernan, C. Kooperberg, et al., "Women's health initiative cohort study," *JAMA* 290 (2003): 1331–1336.

11. H. H. Malluche, N. Koszewski, et al., "Influence of the parathyroid glands on bone metabolism," *European Journal of Clinical Investigation* 36, suppl. 2 (August 2006): 23–33.

12. Kessler, *The Bone Density Program*, 74, 75.

Chapter 5

1. P. Seale, B. Bjork, et al., "PRDM16 controls a brown fat/skeletal muscle switch," *Nature* 454 (August 2008): 961–967.

2. O. B. Cimen, B. Ulba, et al., "Pulmonary function tests, respiratory muscle strength, and endurance of patients with osteoporosis," *Southern Medical Journal* 96, no. 5 (2003): 423–426.

3. S. J. Stear, A. Prentice, et al., "Effect of a calcium and exercise intervention on the bone mineral status of 16–18-year-old adolescent girls," *American Journal of Clinical Nutrition* 77 (2003): 985–992.

4. G. C. Gauchard, P. Gangloff, et al., "Influence of regular proprioceptive and bioenergetic physical activities on balance control in elderly women," *Journals of Gerontology Series A: Biological Sciences and Medical Sciences* 58 (2003): M846–M850.

5. M. L. Irwin, Y. Yasui, et al., "Effect of exercise on total and intra-abdominal body fat in postmenopausal women: A randomized controlled trial," *JAMA* 289 (2003): 323–330.

6. M. Sinaki, R. H. Brey, et al., "Significant reduction in risk of falls and back pain in osteoporotic-kyphotic women through a spinal proprioceptive extension exercise dynamic (SPEED) program," *Mayo Clinic Proceedings* 80, no. 7 (2005): 849–855.

7. N. Miyakoshi, M. Hongo, et al., "Factors related to spinal mobility in patients with postmenopausal osteoporosis," *Osteoporos International* 16, no. 12 (2005): 1871–1874. Sinaki, Brey, et al., "Significant reduction in risk of falls and back pain in osteoporotic-kyphotic women through a spinal proprioceptive extension exercise dynamic (SPEED) program."

8. M. Sinaki, E. Itoi, et al., "Stronger back muscles reduce the incidence of vertebral fractures: A prospective 10 year follow-up of postmenopausal women," *Bone* 30, no. 6 (2002): 836–841. M. Sinaki and B. A. Mikkelsen, "Postmenopausal spinal osteoporosis: Flexion versus extension exercises," *Archives of Physical Medicine and Rehabilitation* 65, no. 10 (October 1984): 593–596. Knut Schmidt-Nielsen, *Scaling: Why Is Animal Size So Important?* (New York: Cambridge University Press, 1984).

Chapter 6

1. J. Wolff, *The Law of Bone Transformation* (Berlin: A. Hirschwald, 1892).

2. P. Forey and P. Janvier, "Evolution of the early vertebrates," *American Scientist* 82 (1994): 554–565. J. D. Jovanović and M. L. Jovanović, "Biomechanical model of vertebra based on bone remodeling," *Medicine and Biology* 11, no. 1 (2004): 35–39.

3. C. T. Rubin, L. E. Lanyon, and G. Baust, "Modulation of bone loss during calcium insufficiency by controlled dynamic load," *Calcified Tissue International* 38 (1986): 209–216.

4. M. J. Pead, R. Suswillo, et al., "Increased 3H-uridine levels in osteocytes following a single short period of dynamic bone loading in vivo," *Calcified Tissue International* 43 (1988): 93–97.

5. C. T. Rubin and L. E. Lanyon, "Regulation of bone formation by applied dynamic loads," *Journal of Bone and Joint Surgery* 66-A (1984): 397–402.

6. C. Kung, "A possible unifying principle for mechanosensation," *Nature* 436, no. 7051 (August 2005): 647–654.

7. Rubin and Lanyon, "Regulation of bone formation by applied dynamic loads."

Chapter 7

1. Y. Li, C. N. Devault, and S. Van Oteghen, "Effects of extended tai chi intervention on balance and selected motor functions of the elderly," *American Journal of Chinese Medicine* 35, no. 3 (2007): 383–391. L. M. Fishman and E. Saltonstall, "Yoga for pain," in *Integrative Pain Medicine: The Science and Practice of Complementary and Alternative Medicine in Pain Management*, ed. Joseph F. Audette and Allison Bailey (Totowa, NJ: Humana Press), 259–284.

2. T. Matsumoto, M. Kawakami, et al., "Cyclic mechanical stretch stress increases the growth rate and collagen synthesis of nucleus pulposus cells in vitro," *Spine* 24, no. 4 (February 1999): 315–319.

3. Weinans and Prendergast, "Adaptation as a dynamical process far from equilibrium."

4. See, for example, the following studies:
   D. C. Cherkin, J. Erro, et al., "Comparing yoga, exercise, and a self-care book for chronic low back pain: A randomized trial," *Annals of Internal Medicine* 143 (2005): 849–856.
   S. Cooper, J. Oborne, et al., "Effect of two breathing exercises (Buteyko and pranayama) in asthma: a randomised controlled trial," *Thorax* 58, no. 8 (August 2003): 674–679.

G. R. Deckro, K. M. Ballinger, et al., "The evaluation of a mind/body intervention to reduce psychological distress and perceived stress in college students," *Journal of American College Health* 50, no. 6 (May 2002): 281–287.

M. DiBenedetto, K. E. Innes, et al., "Effect of a gentle Iyengar yoga program on gait in the elderly: An exploratory study," *Archives of Physical Medicine and Rehabilitation* 86 (September 2005): 1830–1837.

L. M. Fishman and C. Konnoth, "Role of headstand in the management of rotator cuff syndrome," *American Journal of Physical Medicine and Rehabilitation* 83, no. 3 (March 2004): 228, abstract.

L. M. Fishman, C. Konnoth, and A. Polesin, "Headstand for rotator cuff tear: *Sirsasana* or surgery," *Journal of the International Association of Yoga Therapists* 16 (October 2006): 39–46.

M. S. Garfinkel, H. R. Schumacher Jr., et al., "Evaluation of a yoga-based regimen for treatment of osteoarthritis of the hands," *Journal of Rheumatology* 21, no. 12 (December 1994): 2341.

I. Haslock, R. Monro, et al., "Measuring the effects of yoga in rheumatoid arthritis," *British Journal of Rheumatology* 33, no. 8 (August 1994): 787–788.

S. C. Jain, A. Uppal, et al., "A study of response pattern of non-insulin dependent diabetes to yoga therapy," *Diabetes Research and Clinical Practice* 19 (1993): 69–74.

S. L. Kolasinski, A. G. Tsai, et al., "Iyengar yoga for treating symptoms of osteoarthritis of the knees: A pilot study," *Journal of Alternative and Complementary Medicine* 11, no. 4 (August 2005): 689–693.

L. E. Lanyon, "Osteoporosis and exercise," *Topics in Geriatric Rehabilitation* 4, no. 2 (March 1989): 12–24.

S. W. Lazar, C. E. Kerr, et al., "Meditation experience is associated with increased cortical thickness," *Neuroreport* 16, no. 17 (November 2005): 1893–1897.

B. S. Oken, S. Kishiyama, et al., "Randomized controlled trial of yoga and exercise in multiple sclerosis," *Neurology* 62, no. 11 (June 2004): 2058–2064.

C. Peng, I. C. Henry, et al., "Heart rate dynamics during three forms of meditation," *International Journal of Cardiology* 95, no. 1 (May 2004): 19–27.

P. Raghuraj and S. Telles, "Effect of yoga-based and forced uninostril breathing on the autonomic nervous system," *Perceptual and Motor Skills* 96, no. 1 (February 2003): 79–80.

S. Telles, B. H. Hanumanthaiah, et al., "Plasticity of motor control systems demonstrated by yoga training," *Indian Journal of Physiological Pharmacology* 38, no. 2 (April 1994): 143–144.

K. A. Williams, J. Petronis, et al., "Effect of Iyengar yoga therapy for chronic low back pain," *Pain* 115, nos. 1–2 (May 2005):107–117.

A. L. Williams, P. A. Selwyn, et al., "A randomized controlled trial of meditation and massage effects on quality of life in people with late-stage disease: A pilot study," *Journal of Palliative Medicine* 8, no. 5 (October 2005): 939–952.

5. B. K. S. Iyengar, *Light on Yoga* (New York: Schocken Books, 1966), introduction.

Afterword

1. G. F. Anderson and E. Chu, "Expanding priorities: Confronting chronic disease in countries with low income," *New England Journal of Medicine* 356, no. 3 (2006): 209–211.

Resources

Web sites

Anusara-trained teachers:	*www.anusara.com*
Iyengar-trained teachers:	*www.iynaus.org*
Study on yoga and osteoporosis:	*www.sciatica.org*
Loren Fishman:	*www.sciatica.org*
Ellen Saltonstall:	*www.mohiniyoga.com*
Yoga props:	*www.yoga.com* *www.toolsforyoga.com* *www.huggermugger.com*
Morse Fall Scale:	*http://sacramento.networkofcare.org/ library/Morse%20Fall%20Scale.pdf*
Cummings Hip Scale:	*http://cat.inist.fr/?aModele=afficheN& cpsidt=13918533*
Fracture Risk Calculator:	*http://courses.washington.edu/bonephys /Fxriskcalculator.html*

Organizations

American Association of Clinical Endocrinologists
245 Riverside Avenue, Suite 200
Jacksonville, FL 32202
Phone: (904) 353-7878
Web site: www.aace.com

International Association of Yoga Therapists
115 S. McCormick Street, Suite 3
Prescott, AZ 86303
Phone: (928) 541-0004
Web site: www.iayt.org

National Osteoporosis Foundation
1232 22nd Street NW
Washington, DC 20037
Phone: (800) 231-4222
Web site: www.nof.org

North American Menopause Association
P.O. Box 94527
Cleveland, OH 44101
Phone: (440) 442-7550
Web site: www.menopause.org

Magazines

Yoga Journal (www.yogajournal.com)
Yoga + Joyful Living (www.himalayaninstitute.org/yogaplus)

Books

Jeffrey Halter, Joseph Ouslander, Mary Tinetti, and Stephanie Studenski. *Hazzard's Geriatric Medicine & Gerontology,* 6th ed. (New York: McGraw-Hill, 2009). This book is an excellent resource for fall prevention. You may find earlier editions published under the title *Principles of Geriatric Medicine & Gerontology.*

L. C. Junqueira, and J. Carniero. *Basic Histology,* 10th ed. (New York: McGraw-Hill, 2003). If you want to learn about bone tissue and its development, growth, and repair, this is a comprehensive resource.